The Burnout Cure

A Prescription: Romance! Book

JILL BLAKE

ISBN-13: 978-0-9985387-3-0

CONTENTS

CHAPTER ONE

Wolf tapped a finger on the pristine white tablecloth. From across the table, another physician glared at him. Obviously not a fan of syncopated rhythm. Wolf sighed, dropped his hand, and feigned interest in what the hospital's chief of staff was saying.

Another five minutes of the man's rambling welcome speech, and Wolf was back to tapping, this time against his jean-clad thigh.

He should have just stayed in bed. Or gone for a run. Or ironed out the lyrics he'd been toying with for weeks. Or done any of a dozen other things, instead of wasting his Saturday morning listening to a bunch of self-proclaimed experts pontificate about physician wellness.

What the fuck was that, anyway?

The stupid catch phrase seemed to be popping up everywhere. Kind of like *physician burnout*. Another term-of-the-moment Wolf hated. You'd think people would tire of the topic. But no. Whenever he opened a medical journal, or stepped into the doctors' lounge, or went to the ER to admit a patient, there was always someone talking about wellness, burnout, or both.

And now, thanks to his best friend, Wolf had to sit through

1

six more hours of torture. Unless he managed to sneak out early, during one of the breaks. He glanced at the printed itinerary, searching for the two names he'd been assigned. The first was easy enough to find. Lily Reid, the keynote speaker. But the second....He scanned the list to the very end. Yeah, it figured. The last speaker of the day.

He was going to kill Doug for getting him into this.

Of course, it wasn't Doug's fault that his wife went into premature labor last night. But the guy could have tried a little harder to find someone else to sub for him. Someone who wasn't Wolf. Someone who actually *chose* to serve on Doug's damn committee. What was the point of being chair if you couldn't delegate scut work to other committee members, rather than dumping it on your best friend?

"Come on, man," Doug had said over the phone, after waking Wolf from the first decent sleep he'd had in week. "Free food, six hours of CME credit, and you'll be out of there by one at the latest."

"You've got to be kidding me," Wolf groaned. "No amount of free food is worth sitting through six hours of BS."

Doug sighed. "Just because you've got the sensibility of a rhinoceros doesn't make the issue any less real or important."

"Give me a break," Wolf said. In the background, he could hear the familiar sounds of the hospital: a monitor beeping, the low murmur of voices. "It's one in the morning. You really want to debate this? Now?"

"Two introductions," Doug said. "A minute each. That's all I'm asking."

Wolf rubbed his eyes and leaned back against the headboard. "Don't you have someone else you can tap?"

"Like you said, bro, it's one in the morning. Everyone else has a spouse or family. You know, a life."

"Fuck you," Wolf said. "I have a life—"

A sharp cry on the other end of the line cut him off.

"Gotta go," Doug said, "I'll email you the text."

And that was how Wolf ended up at the 65th Annual Postgraduate Medical Assembly, waiting to introduce some quack hired by the hospital to explain how to get in touch with your inner child. Or whatever motivational mumbo-jumbo the woman planned to sell as the latest antidote to burnout.

Applause rippled through the hotel ballroom. Wolf glanced around the half-occupied tables. A few late arrivals trickled in, armed with coffee and pastries from the continental breakfast just outside.

Wolf reached for his own mug. Empty. Crap. Was there time to slip out for a refill? The applause petered out before he could take a step toward the exit. And then the chief of staff was talking again, and it was too late.

"Ladies and gentlemen," the man said, "I'd like to introduce the chair of our Physician Health Committee, who is also the head of St. Mary's Pulmonary and Critical Care department, Dr. Douglas Williams."

Wolf checked the pocket of his sport coat for the notes he'd printed out earlier. Still there. Okay, then. Showtime.

The smattering of applause dwindled amid whispers and laughter as he approached the podium. The chief of staff raised his brows.

"Sorry." Wolf offered him a smile and handshake, then gestured toward the microphone. "May I?"

The man scanned the crowd, then shot Wolf a warning look before stepping back. What, did he expect Wolf to hijack the meeting? Inject some off-color humor into the proceedings? Sure, the thought had crossed Wolf's mind. But prankster reputation or not, he had no desire to prolong what already promised to be a long, painful day.

"As some of you may have noticed, I'm not Dr. Williams," he began. "My name is Wolf Knox, and I'm a hospitalist. For anyone who's been living under a rock for the last decade or so, a hospitalist is the guy who takes care of your patients while they're overnight guests at St. Mary's. Now you're probably asking yourself: *why am I here today?* Putting aside the existential question—because I hear they're kicking us out of this room at one p.m., ready or not—the reason I'm here at this podium is because Doug asked me to step in while he's off having a baby—"

"Doug's pregnant?" someone called out from a back table.

Wolf waited for the laughter to die down. "I stand corrected. Doug's wife was the one who went into labor last night. So while Doug and the missus are busy ushering in the next generation of Williamses, I'm going to introduce a few folks who've traveled a long way to talk to you today. You ready? All loaded up on caffeine? Feeling a bit jittery from all that java? Well, don't worry. Our keynote speaker is here to share her secrets about relaxation. Which, for those of you keeping track of this sort of thing, is the keyword of the day. Come on, folks, say it with me. *Reee-laaax-aaa-tion*. Oh, and don't forget to sign up for the free yoga and meditation session in the courtyard after lunch."

From the corner of his eye, Wolf caught a glimpse of the chief of staff's frown.

Uh-oh. Maybe he'd gone too far.

Wolf cleared his throat. "Sorry, folks, looks like the yoga session's been canceled. The Physician Health Committee will work on getting it rescheduled, once Dr. Williams returns from paternity leave. In the meantime, please help me welcome Dr. Lily Reid, who comes to us straight from a sold-out engagement on the lecture circuit. In case you're wondering why Dr. Reid is so popular, here's the twenty-second version of her CV."

He retrieved Doug's notes from his pocket and smoothed out the creases. "Dr. Reid received her medical degree and Master of Public Health from UCSD. She joined the RAND Corporation seven years ago, where she is now a research fellow in healthcare policy. Her articles on health and wellness have been published in top medical journals as well as the lay press, and she is a regular talking head—uh, guest—on radio and cable TV news. Please put your hands together for Dr. Lily Reid."

A flurry of movement along the far wall caught Wolf's attention.

Hot damn. *This* was Lily Reid?

She wore a pencil skirt that ended just above the knee, a white button-down shirt, and a black belt that emphasized her narrow waist. With her auburn hair slicked back into a neat bun, a single strand of pearls around her neck, and those red, red lips, she was the embodiment of every sexy librarian fantasy he'd had as an adolescent.

He grinned, watching as she wound her way between tables toward the front. The skirt pulled tight across her hips with each step. When she reached the podium and turned to face the audience, Wolf's eyes dropped to her rounded ass.

Oh, yeah. Some fantasies just got better with age.

She adjusted the microphone and glanced up at him, catching the direction of his gaze. Dark green eyes narrowed, and her mouth tightened. For a moment his brain short-circuited as he pictured those lips doing wicked things to his anatomy.

She cleared her throat. "Thank you for that...colorful...introduction."

Ouch. Baby had claws.

His grin widened and he leaned in. Ignoring her quick intake of breath, he plucked his notes from the lectern and pocketed them. "All yours, Doc."

By the time he sauntered back to his seat, she'd already launched into her presentation.

Work-life balance. Physical and spiritual energy. The dangers of sleep deprivation, overwork, eroding compassion.

Oh, man. The fun was definitely over.

Wolf fished out his phone. At least the cell reception was decent. That was the first thing he'd checked on arriving. If nothing else, he'd catch up on email. Scroll through the digital edition of today's *L.A. Times*. Maybe shoot a few zombies, though it wouldn't be as much fun with the sound effects off.

A glance around the room confirmed he wasn't the only one looking to his phone for entertainment. What surprised him was how many people appeared to be listening with rapt attention, even nodding in agreement with whatever point Lily Reid was making.

He looked toward the front.

She was pacing now, slashing the air with one hand, holding the microphone in the other.

"...highest suicide rate of any profession. We lose four hundred physicians a year to suicide. That's more than an entire medical school class. *Every year...*"

Seriously, could she have picked a more depressing topic?

He tuned out the words, focusing instead on the way she looked. Fierce. Intense. Passionate.

Oh, yeah. He wouldn't mind exploring some of that passion. Seeing what it would take to get her to loosen up, let down her hair, undo a few more of those buttons.

Suddenly his day was looking up. All he had to do was stick it out until the talks were done, and then make his move.

There were so many people milling about after the final Q&A session that Wolf almost missed seeing her slip out through a side door.

He rushed after her, his long strides narrowing the distance between them.

"Hey, Doc," he said, when he finally caught up to her in the hotel lobby. "Nice talk."

She glanced up at him and blinked. "Thanks. Dr....?"

"Knox," he said, trying not to feel slighted. "But you can call me Wolf."

She nodded and continued toward the exit. Wolf kept pace with her.

"Did you even hear a word I said?" she asked, when it became clear that he wasn't going away.

"Of course," Wolf said. "Every word."

Oh, yeah, she'd noticed him. Enough to comment on his inattention. Which begged the question: had she really forgotten his name, or had that been a deliberate dig, too?

A uniformed attendant opened the door, and they stepped into the afternoon heat.

"Every word. Right." Lily slanted him a look before pulling a pair of sunglasses from her computer bag. "So what did you think about the documentary idea?"

Wolf paused in the process of donning his own sunglasses. "Uh…brilliant?"

"Nice try."

He trailed after her toward the parking valet stand. Several conference attendees were already clustered there, chatting as they waited for their cars.

One of the men broke off from the crowd and approached her with a smile. "John Hunter," he said, offering a handshake. "I'm an orthopedist at St. Mary's."

She nodded. "Nice to meet you."

Instead of relinquishing her hand, Hunter stepped closer. "So, Lily—you don't mind if I call you Lily? How long will you be in town?"

Wolf scowled and moved to her side. "Hunter. How's that fiancée of yours?"

The guy dropped Lily's hand. "Fine," he said. "By the way, Wolfman, she wanted to pass along her compliments. Said you look good in drag."

Wolf's eyes flickered to Lily. She stared back, brows raised. Great. Now she thought he was a cross-dresser. Or gay. Or *something* that required explanation.

"Well, this is me," Hunter said, as the valet pulled up in a flashy convertible. "It's been a pleasure, Lily. Hope to see you around."

Lily watched as he slid behind the wheel and peeled away from the curb.

"Forget him," Wolf growled. "He's an asshole. Hits on all the nurses."

"Of course he does," she murmured. "And I'm sure he's not the only one."

Wolf started to offer a rebuttal, then thought better of it. He wasn't a hypocrite. Sure, he didn't have a fiancée like Hunter did. And if a woman didn't respond to flirtation, Wolf backed off. Okay, maybe not now, but usually.

Another car pulled up. Wolf eyed the dwindling crowd. Any minute, one of the valets would ask for their tickets.

Now or never.

"Let's have lunch," Wolf said, "and you can tell me more about this documentary."

"They served lunch at the conference."

"Yeah, but you didn't eat."

Her mouth fell open. "How…?"

"I was watching you," he said. "So what do you say? I know this great tapas place…"

"Sorry." She glanced at her watch. "I need to get to the airport."

"Oh. When's your flight?"

She hesitated. "It's a red-eye. But I still need to get home to shower and pack."

A fresh wave of conference attendees spilled out onto the street.

Wolf cupped Lily's elbow and urged her out of the way, nodding to the new arrivals to cut ahead.

Lily frowned, but before she could protest, Wolf let go and distracted her. "Where do you live?"

"Why?"

"I'll make sure you get there in plenty of time," he said. "After lunch."

She shook her head. "I don't even know you. Why would I want to have lunch with you?"

"So you can get to know me."

"Look—" she broke off and took a deep breath. "I'm sure you're a perfectly nice person—"

"My mother certainly thinks so."

She smiled. For maybe half a second. If he hadn't been paying such close attention, he would have missed it.

Stubborn female.

The last time he'd had to work this hard for a date was…uh…never. Women loved him. Tall, dark, and handsome might be a cliché, but it worked for him. That, and the "MD" after his name. Feminism hadn't completely erased the allure of marrying a doctor, and some women refused to believe that he wasn't interested in settling down. They thought he was joking. Or maybe they saw his attitude as a challenge.

Whatever. This was the one topic he never joked about. Sex, politics, religion? All fair game. But his personal independence? Hell, no. Not in this lifetime.

He loved being single. Loved the endless all-you-can-eat buffet of femininity, with a different size and shape and color for every mood and taste. Loved having the freedom to push away from the table after gorging himself, and then going home to his own space, where he was accountable to no one, and responsible only for himself.

Lily's voice pulled him back to the moment. "Are you always this persistent?"

"Nah," he said. "I'm pretty laid back. Except when I really want something."

"And now you really want to have lunch."

"With you," he said. In case she'd somehow missed that part.

She bit her lip, drawing his attention to her mouth. Her lipstick had worn off earlier, leaving behind a softer, more vulnerable look. Straight white teeth sank into her lower lip, and he watched, mesmerized. He could almost feel those teeth nipping at his own flesh, her lips and tongue following to soothe the sting. A flash of heat streaked through his body, arrowing straight down to his groin. Sweat that had nothing to do with the afternoon sun beaded along his hairline. Beneath the light-weight sport coat, his T-shirt stuck to his skin. He'd have to start shedding layers if she didn't say something soon. Or better yet, succumb to temptation and swoop in for a taste of those luscious lips.

He was seconds away from doing something stupid when she spoke. "I can forward you a one-page synopsis…"

What? Oh, right, the documentary.

He took a deep breath and blew it out slowly. "I'd be happy to read it. After we do lunch."

She chewed her lip some more. "Fine."

Who knew such a tiny word could unleash such strong emotion? Relief, triumph, and anticipation surged through him.

"Great. I'll drive." Wolf ushered her toward the valet stand, bypassing a handful of curious colleagues. "We can pick up your car later."

"Hold on." She dug a phone out of her bag.

A sudden, unwelcome thought crossed his mind. Just because he was a free agent didn't mean she was. Sure, she wasn't wearing a ring. He made sure of that right after introducing her, once he'd managed to tear his eyes away from her curves. But the absence of a ring didn't negate the possibility of a husband and three kids stashed at home.

He cleared his throat. "Lily."

"Hmm?" She kept her eyes on the screen as she typed.

"What are you doing?"

"Texting a friend." She glanced up. "In case I end up missing. At least the police will know who to look for."

He blinked. She was kidding. Wasn't she? And what exactly did she mean by *friend*?

"There." She put her phone away. "Now we can go."

CHAPTER TWO

Lily tightened her white-knuckle grip on the passenger door armrest. Thank goodness she'd skipped lunch, otherwise the contents of her stomach would be decorating the upholstery by now. "Can you please slow down?"

Wolf swerved around yet another car, like an Indy 500 driver intent on beating the competition.

"Wolf." She swallowed and concentrated on her breathing. "Please. Just pick a lane and stay there."

"What?" He glanced at her. "Oh, hell. You need me to pull over?"

"No." She clenched her teeth. "Just. Slow. Down."

"Right. Sorry." He eased off the gas pedal. "You should have told me you get carsick."

"I don't. Except when someone drives like a maniac."

"It's L.A.," he said. "Everyone drives like a maniac."

"Not me." She loosened her hold on the door just enough to relieve the cramping in her fingers.

"Okay," he conceded. "Almost everyone. Where'd you grow up?"

"Santa Monica."

"Really?" He shot her an assessing look before turning his attention back to the road. "I wouldn't have pegged you for a local."

"Why not?"

"Well, for one thing, people here are used to traffic."

"I'm used to it," she said. "I just don't like it."

"No one likes it. You just learn to deal with it." He covered her hand with a large, warm palm, lightly squeezing her fingers. "Hang on—"

That was all the warning she got. A moment later, they were crossing two lanes of traffic to turn left, barely making it through the intersection before the light turned red.

Oh, God. She squeezed her eyes shut. They were going to die. She wasn't ready to die. She still had too much to do. Workshops to run. Talks to give. A message to spread.

People relied on her, dammit. Lives were at stake.

She gulped and forced her eyes open.

They were on a side street now, slowing down. Pulling into a parking spot.

"We're here," he said. "You can let go now."

She blinked and followed his gaze. "Oh."

Flushing, she released his hand. The one she'd been clutching like a lifeline. It took her trembling fingers a few tries to undo the seatbelt.

"Doing okay?" he said.

She smoothed the wrinkles from her skirt and lifted her chin. "On the way back, I'm driving."

He laughed, setting off a strange fluttering in her belly. As if they were moving again. Even though the car hadn't budged since he'd set it in park.

She pressed a hand against her stomach. Wolf got out, and she watched him walk around the hood of the car.

Ordinarily she wouldn't have waited. She was used to opening her own doors. But she needed a moment to pull herself together. Plus, it gave her the chance to drink in some of the details she'd failed to notice before. Like how tall he was. And well-built.

Oh, hell, who was she kidding? She'd noticed. But at the podium and later, outside the hotel, she'd been too annoyed by his attitude to truly appreciate the physical package.

Now, she couldn't help but admire the six feet of male perfection wrapped in dark fitted jeans, white crew-neck T-shirt, and caramel-colored sport coat. Muscles rippled beneath his clothes as he stepped onto the sidewalk and approached the passenger door.

Where was the paunch that went along with a sedentary lifestyle and crap diet? The pasty skin that attested to endless days spent beneath fluorescent hospital lights?

Her gaze swept over the firm jaw peppered with dark stubble, the tanned neck and broad chest, the lean waist and powerful thighs. She'd seen professional athletes in worse shape.

Maybe St. Mary's had a gym where the staff could burn off excess stress and calories between shifts. Because even if he'd won the genetics lottery, no man could possibly look like Wolf without putting at least some effort into maintenance.

Too soon, the car door opened and a large masculine hand appeared beside her. She placed her palm in his, and inhaled sharply at the tingling sensation that started at the point of contact. She'd been too terrified by his driving to feel it before. Now it was impossible to ignore. His fingers closed over hers, pulling her up. She stumbled slightly, brushing against his chest before his other hand steadied her.

"Okay?" he said.

She nodded, too aware of his proximity, and the faint woodsy smell of his cologne to muster any other response. He reached past her for the computer bag she'd left behind. Instead of handing it over, he shouldered it and closed the door. Then he reclaimed her hand, not letting go until they were inside the restaurant, seated at a rustic wooden table in the corner.

"Something to drink?" the waiter asked.

Lily fumbled for the menu. "Water, please."

"Sure you don't want something stronger?" Wolf said. "The Sangria here is amazing. And I'm driving."

She frowned. "I thought we agreed that I'd drive."

"Sorry," he said. "But that baby was my first big purchase out of residency."

"I'll be extra careful."

He shook his head. "How about this. I promise to go slowly, and you'll at least try the wine."

She checked the time. "It's not even two o'clock. Water's fine."

"Stubborn," he said with a mock sigh.

"Smart," she retorted.

"You win," he grinned. "Water it is. Pellegrino?"

"Yes."

"Two Pellegrinos," he told the waiter. "One Sangria. And we'll need a few minutes."

Lily opened the menu. While pretending to examine her tapas choices, she surreptitiously studied Wolf's bent head and broad shoulders.

She ought to be annoyed with him. Arrogance was usually a huge turn off. And Wolf, without question, had it in spades. Along with impatience and a hefty dose of impudence.

Despite that, something about him intrigued and unsettled her. Enough to push her into behaving impulsively. The pretext of discussing her pet project was just that, a flimsy excuse for accepting his invitation to lunch. She doubted he was any more interested in her ideas now than he had been at the conference, when she'd caught him fidgeting every time she looked his way.

"So where are you headed this evening?" he said, startling her out of her introspection.

She set aside the menu. "Boston."

"For business or pleasure?"

"Business. I'm running a three-day physician retreat on finding meaning in medicine." His burst of laughter had her frowning. "What's so funny?"

"Sorry. It's just—*three days*? I can tell you the meaning in three *words*. Treat. Sick. Patients." He ticked off each word with his fingers. "Or how about this? Keep. Patients. Healthy."

"From a patient's perspective, you're probably right," she

said. "But as a doctor, is that really enough to get you out of bed and into the hospital each morning?"

"Sure," he said. "And the steady paycheck doesn't hurt either."

"Seriously?" She raised a brow. "That's enough to compensate for all the time and energy you waste dealing with stupid bureaucracy? All the insurance companies, regulatory agencies, career administrators who micromanage everything you do? They know less about medicine than your average pre-med student, but they still have the power to overrule your best clinical judgment and dictate how you treat patients."

"Of course I don't *love* it," he said. "But I do my best to ignore it."

"You can't ignore it if it's mandated as quality improvement. Or pay for performance. Or whatever the bureaucrats are calling it these days."

"Okay, so it's not perfect," he shrugged. "Nothing is. But you don't see me sitting around all day, complaining."

"No, of course not," she said. "You'd rather sit at the computer all day, clicking their 'meaningful use' boxes, like some glorified data entry clerk with the courtesy title of doctor."

"Ouch." He winced. "You must be familiar with our EMR."

"It's not just yours. Almost every physician I talk to has horror stories about their electronic medical record. And the rest have either given up clinical practice, or invested in scribes."

"Fine," he said. "You've made your point. I assume you have a solution. Or do I have to sign up for one of your retreats to hear it?"

Like that was ever going to happen. She couldn't see him lasting through a single day of panel discussions and mindfulness exercises, let alone three.

"It's all about stress management," she said. "Replacing self-destructive behaviors with healthier ways of managing stress."

The laugh lines around his eyes crinkled. "Like yoga?"

"Smirk all you want," she said. "But it actually works. I can send you links to dozens of studies that show how yoga lowers blood pressure and heart rate, improves sleep, reduces inflammatory markers—"

He raised his palms in surrender. "Okay, I believe you. Personally I prefer surfing, but to each his own."

She swallowed. Well, that accounted for the tan. She could picture him bare-chested in low-riding board shorts, skin gleaming with droplets of water, muscles flexing as he rode the waves. There was no room in her fantasy for rash guards or skin suits, even though logic—and the perpetually cold waters off the Santa Monica and Malibu coast—dictated that most surfers cover up.

Their waiter returned, opening the trademark green bottle and pouring sparkling water into two tall glasses. "Ready to order?"

She picked up her discarded menu and glanced at Wolf. "You go first."

He rattled off a list of dishes while Lily skimmed her choices.

"So," Wolf said, after the waiter left with their orders, "that's all it takes to bring a disgruntled physician back into the fold? Three days of yoga?"

"No." She smoothed the napkin across her lap. "Yoga's just an example. One of the many things that can help improve work-life balance. It can be anything, really. Mountain climbing. Knitting. Joining a book club. Doing karaoke."

"Having sex?"

His voice stroked across her skin, leaving goosebumps in its wake. Images of tangled limbs and heated bodies—his and hers—flickered through her head.

She blinked. No. Absolutely not. This might be the longest dry spell she'd experienced since going off to college, but there was no way she was jumping into bed with a virtual stranger. Bad enough she'd agreed to have lunch with him. But getting naked? Not happening.

She lifted her chin. "Like I said, any activity that reminds us there's more to life than work. That's the key. By cultivating outside interests, we can put things in perspective. That's what allows us to look beyond the daily frustrations and regain our sense of purpose. In other words, rediscover whatever motivated us to go into medicine in the first place."

He took a sip of Sangria. "Interesting theory."

"You're not convinced."

"No offense, Lily." He set the glass down. "But it seems odd that all these docs would look to you for advice about— what'd you call it, finding meaning in medicine?"

"Why does it seem odd?"

"Because you quit medicine after a year of internship. That doesn't exactly make you an expert." He cocked a brow. "Unless I misread your CV?"

Wolf wasn't the first to question her credentials. Years of fielding similar criticism had almost inured her to it. But the condescending tone, coming on the heels of his earlier flirtation? *That* stung.

"No," she finally said. "You didn't misread it. But I did graduate med school. And a year of internship is no walk in the park."

"True," he said. "But—"

"Personal experience," she interrupted, "isn't the only—or necessarily the best—qualification for the type of work I do. I've spent hundreds of hours interviewing doctors at various stages of their careers, gathering data on how stressors affect job performance, family life, anxiety and depression scores. I've written papers and policy statements, testified before various commissions on graduate medical education. I could go on, but the bottom line is I've seen how brutal things can get. The hazing and abuse of doctors-in-training is so entrenched that it's considered normal. And it doesn't stop with residency, especially for women. We're taught to take it and keep our mouths shut. If we dare complain or show any sign of weakness, we might as well kiss our careers goodbye."

His gaze sharpened. "Is that what happened to you?"

"No." She swallowed against the rising tide of pain and anger that still sometimes threatened to choke her. "I guess I was lucky. But there were others around me who…weren't."

"And that's why you quit? Someone you knew failed, so you decided it wasn't worth the effort to continue? Or were you afraid you couldn't hack it?"

The words echoed her father's so closely that she had to take a deep breath and blow it out slowly before answering.

Seven years after the fact, she could still hear her father's voice shaking as he threatened to disown her. *Reids are not quitters*, he'd railed. *You will pull yourself together and finish what you started.*

But by then she'd already embarked on a new path. Her temporary leave of absence from residency turned into a permanent change of career. And unlike medicine, which she'd only pursued because it was expected of her, this new career became her *raison d'être*. Her salvation during the darkest moments of her life, the one thing she could cling to and count on when everything else was lost.

She met Wolf's gaze head-on. "I made a conscious decision to switch tracks. Do something that I felt could make a real difference."

"Of course," he nodded. "There aren't enough yoga teachers around."

She ignored his sarcasm. "My research at RAND allows me to shine a light on the real-world challenges doctors face every day. That's the first step in fixing any broken system. You need to identify and document the problems."

Their food arrived, putting a halt to the conversation.

"Another Sangria, sir?" the waiter asked.

"No, thanks. But we could use some more water."

They ate in silence. The waiter returned with another bottle of Pellegrino and topped off both their glasses.

Wolf waited until they were alone again to resume their conversation. "Does RAND sponsor your workshops?"

"No. That's something I do on my own."

He paused, fork suspended halfway between his mouth and

plate. "Why?"

"Because change doesn't happen overnight, and papers and policy statements only get you so far. There are lots of people out there who can't wait a year or two or ten for things to improve. Physicians who feel trapped and can't see their way out, who've devoted so much time and energy to taking care of others that they've neglected to take care of themselves. They need help now, before they decide to do something drastic that can't be undone."

"Like what?" he said. "Quit medicine?"

"Or commit suicide." She met his gaze, almost daring him to say something derisive.

He didn't. Instead, he set down his utensils and wiped his mouth with a napkin. "You want to know what I think?"

She hesitated. "Sure."

"Medicine's not for everyone," he said. "You can be smart and hardworking and ace the boards on your first try. But if being a doctor stresses you out so much that you'd consider suicide...baby, you're in the wrong field."

Her fingers tightened around her glass. For a moment, she imagined dumping the contents over his head. Maybe he'd be a little less judgmental with ice water dripping down his nose. "In other words," she said, "your litmus test for whether someone's worthy of being a doctor is whether or not they're depressed."

"Well, obviously there are other criteria too," he said. "But yes, people with depression—or any mental illness that can affect their cognitive ability and judgment—should be weeded out."

"Wow. Do you even know how many medical students and residents that would affect?"

"No. But I guess you're going to tell me?"

"Thirty percent."

He narrowed his eyes. "I don't believe it."

She shrugged. "The statistics speak for themselves."

"What statistics?"

"Results from two big meta-analyses published in *JAMA*.

One on medical students, the other on residents. They pooled data from some two hundred studies looking at prevalence of depression. It made a huge splash in the lay press as well." She raised a brow. "I take it you missed the coverage?"

"I must have been working that day."

She pursed her lips. "There's more—"

"You're kidding."

"No, that was just about med students and docs-in-training," she said. "Let's talk about your colleagues."

"What about them?"

"*Medscape* publishes a yearly physician lifestyle report. Fourteen thousand physicians across various specialties surveyed, and over fifty percent admit to feeling burned out."

He groaned. "Not that again."

"Excuse me?"

"Burnout." He wrinkled his nose, as if he'd just smelled something foul. "What a crock. Those surveys you're quoting are totally skewed. You realize that, don't you? Disgruntled physicians are more likely to fill out some questionnaire about their grievances than those of us who are busy working in the trenches."

"The authors adjust for non-participation bias—"

"Let me tell you something." He pushed aside his plate and leaned forward, resting his arms on the table. "Being a doctor isn't supposed to be easy. Or convenient. Anyone who's made it *all the way* through med school and residency knows that. You're dealing with people's lives, and that's a huge responsibility. Doesn't matter if you're sleep-deprived, and you've been on your feet all day, and you've already rounded on thirty patients—if the ER calls with a new admission, you suck it up and do your job. That's what you signed up for when you decided to become a doctor. So instead of preaching about yoga and mountain climbing, maybe you should tell all those so-called burned-out physicians to stop bitching and moaning about the hours and the workload and simply follow your example. Don't like it? Can't hack it? Do everyone a favor and get the hell out of medicine."

Lily clenched her fists in her lap, nails digging into her palms. He might as well have reached across the table and slapped her.

Smug. Narrow-minded. Bastard.

But angry as she was at him, she was even angrier at herself.

He, at least, had been consistent, dropping clues from the very start. The irreverent introduction. The fidgeting during her talk. The steady flow of patronizing questions and snide remarks. Sure, he'd managed to disguise some of it as humor. But now even the pretense of affability wore off.

She should have stuck with her first instinct and refused his invitation to lunch. Instead, she'd allowed his looks and flirtation to lull her into ignoring the voice of reason.

Well, enough of that. She had a mile-long list of things she had to do before heading for the airport. Time to get on with it.

Looking around, she spied her computer bag propped against the wall beside Wolf's chair. Out of her reach, unless she crawled beneath the table. Or asked him to hand it over.

She glanced up, but the words died in her throat. He was watching her, his brown eyes so dark they were almost black. Her lips parted, and his gaze dropped to her mouth.

Their waiter returned, breaking the tension. "How are you doing, folks? Can I get you anything else?"

"No," Lily said, shaking off the odd torpor that had taken hold of her limbs. "Thank you."

"Maybe some coffee?" the man asked. "Or a dessert menu? We have a *quesada pasiega* that's very light. And you can't go wrong with the flan—"

"Just the check," Wolf interrupted. "Thank you."

"Very good, sir."

They waited in strained silence while he cleared the table and withdrew, Wolf's credit card tucked into a black leather bill holder beneath his arm.

"Look," Wolf said. "I'm sorry if I offended you."

Lily folded her napkin and placed it on the table. His apology was almost as insulting as his earlier diatribe. "Thank you for lunch."

"We never got around to discussing that documentary you mentioned."

"No."

"I have time this afternoon—"

"I don't," she said. "If you'll hand me my bag, I can take an Uber back to the hotel."

He didn't move. "I'll drive you."

Lily bit her lip. "I'm not sure my stomach can handle your driving."

His smile, even now, even after everything he'd said, had the power to spike her pulse. "I'll go nice and slow. Promise."

If she didn't have a flight to catch…

If he weren't such a stubborn, egotistical jerk…

If she were a little less principled…

The waiter returned. Wolf finished taking care of the bill, picked up Lily's bag, and rose. "Ready?"

He rested his hand on the small of her back as they made their way toward the exit. Heat, completely at odds with her mood, spread through her body. And that damn flutter was back.

She thought about protesting. Pulling away. But what difference would another minute or two make? His car was right outside. A short ride back to the hotel, and she'd never have to see him again.

He drew to a halt beside the passenger door. "You're back Tuesday?"

"Wednesday."

He nodded and ushered her inside. True to his word, he stayed in the slow lane. Before she knew it, they were pulling up to the hotel, and a valet approached to open her door.

Wolf caught her hand before she had a chance to get out. "I'll call you."

Later, as she sat in the window seat doing a final read-through of tomorrow's opening presentation on her laptop, Wolf's promise echoed in her head.

She hadn't given him her number, and he hadn't asked for

it.

An oversight? Or had he meant the words as a pleasantry, to draw their disagreement to a polite close?

Either way, did it matter? She had no interest in pursuing anything with Wolf. Even if he did manage to find her contact information online and call.

Sure, he was attractive. Intelligent. Funny—even if some of that humor stung.

But he was also an unapologetic chauvinist. Like her father. Like so many old-school physicians whose *suck it up or get the hell out* machismo perpetuated the abuses in medical education and practice. The abuses she's spent the past seven years fighting.

Was she really prepared to chuck her principles out the window just because her long-dead libido had chosen this moment to stir back to life?

She pushed the question aside. No point worrying over hypothetical problems. *If* Wolf called, she'd reassess the situation.

Until then, she had work to do.

CHAPTER THREE

Flu season might be off to a slow start, at least according to the CDC, but the hospital census at St. Mary's sure didn't reflect that. Wolf had five new admissions before the ER went on divert, and of the other eighteen patients he rounded on, only two were stable enough for discharge. The topper, though, came toward the end of the day, when one of his heart failure patients coded. For a while it was touch and go, but thankfully they managed to get the guy stabilized and transferred to the ICU.

By the time Wolf finished hand-off to the night team, his twelve hours had dragged into fourteen. The hospital cafeteria was long closed, and the limited vending machine options held little appeal. Wolf tried to remember if he had anything edible in his fridge at home. Probably not. The last time he'd gone food shopping was two—or was it three?—weeks ago.

Good thing his favorite Chinese takeout place was open late.

A quick shower and change of clothes in the call room, and he headed out, scrolling through phone messages as he strode down the hall toward the main lobby.

A text from Doug: *All well, now home. Tina says thx for flowers.*

He should probably drop by next week when he was off.

See the little guy who was indirectly responsible for his latest obsession.

Or maybe obsession was too strong a word. Preoccupation? Fascination? Infatuation?

In the three days since meeting Lily and sparring with her over lunch, Wolf found his thoughts returning to her time and again. Picturing the way her eyes flashed when she disagreed with him. Feeling the visceral tug of desire whenever those teeth worried her lower lip. Wondering what would have happened if they'd followed the usual getting-to-know-you script instead of veering off into a discussion of work that turned out to be strewn with conversational landmines.

Last night he'd looked her up online. Damn, the woman got around. The sheer number and variety of past speaking engagements on her website might have intimidated a lesser man. But Wolf skimmed right past them to the contact information. The number took him to an automated phone tree. He followed the voice prompts for *all other inquiries* and left a message with his cell number.

If she didn't call back…well, he'd give it a few days before trying again.

He tapped on the phone icon and checked missed calls. First up was a voicemail from a number he didn't recognize.

Hi Wolf, it's Cathy. I know it's short notice—

He frowned. Who the hell was Cathy?

—a few of us are heading over to O' Briens and I was wondering if maybe you'd like to come—

Ah, that Cathy. The cute little scrub nurse he'd hooked up with a couple weeks ago. The one with perky tits and the most amazing lasagna he'd ever tasted. A family recipe, she said, made from scratch. Shit, he'd promised to call her, hadn't he?

—Anyway, it's seven-forty and we'll probably hang out another hour or two, so stop by if you want.

O'Briens was two blocks north of the hospital. She was probably still there. A week ago, he might have considered walking over.

But she didn't have eyes the color of a Douglas fir. Her

opinions—when they'd taken a break for food and conversation—seemed about as profound and controversial as watery Cream of Wheat. And frankly, he didn't relish repeat performances. Even if they came with the promise of home-cooked lasagna.

He'd send her a box of chocolates with a note. *Sorry and best wishes.* Or something like that. No point in being an asshole, but he didn't want to encourage her either. Not with his head and libido all wrapped up in another woman.

Next message. Some telemarketer offering him a discount cruise to Alaska.

Delete.

His mother calling to remind him about his nephew's birthday party. He paused to do a quick online search-and-order. He'd given up trying to keep track of his nieces' and nephews' mercurial taste in toys and gadgets. Whatever the kid wanted, Wolf had no doubt that Amazon carried it. There. One electronic gift card on its way.

A quick swipe through his email inbox revealed nothing urgent.

Wolf pocketed the phone, zipped up his leather jacket, and loped down the stairs toward the staff parking lot.

"Hi there, Dr. Knox," the attendant said. "Heard there's rain in the forecast. Be careful on the road."

"Thanks, Ramon," Wolf said. "See you tomorrow."

By the time her flight landed at LAX on Wednesday afternoon, Lily was ready to crawl into bed and stay there. The workshops left her physically and emotionally drained. Too many physicians in crisis. She couldn't reach, let alone save, all of them. Logically, she understood that. But it didn't make the knowledge or guilt any easier to bear.

As the plane taxied toward the gate, she pulled out her phone. Five missed calls.

The first, from her best friend Parker, made her smile.

"Hey, Lil," he said. "I found a new place. The Lumberyard Tavern, in Encinitas. Two pounds of beef, four strips of bacon, four slices of cheese, fried egg, pretzel dough bun. Optional lettuce, tomato, and onion. Text me if you're game and we'll meet there Saturday."

One of these days, his heart-attack-on-a-plate diet would catch up with him, and no amount of running was going to save him. Whenever she told him that, Parker would counter, "You gotta loosen up and live a little."

Lily texted him: *Yes @ noon. Bring the Wiggs file.*

He responded immediately with a thumbs-up and address.

There were two hang-ups, then a reminder from her administrative assistant about the back-to-back meetings she had tomorrow, starting at eight.

Lily sighed. She'd spent most of the flight on her computer, prepping, and would likely need another four to five hours once she got home.

The last call was the one she'd been hoping for—and dreading.

"Lily, it's Wolf." His voice was warm, intimate. "Hope your retreat went well. I'm on service this week, but should be off Friday night. How does dinner at eight sound? I was thinking Thai, unless you had something else in mind. Call me."

Did she want to see Wolf again? Her pulse spiked. A kaleidoscope of butterflies took up residence in her belly. Oh, yeah.

But did seeing him mean she had to suffer through another meal, defending her convictions? Maybe if they stuck with neutral topics, it wouldn't be so bad. Or they could skip dinner altogether. What was food anyway, other than foreplay, dressed up in pretty clothes? Why not strip away all the social niceties and simply acknowledge what they both wanted?

The more she thought about it on the way home from the airport, the more it made sense.

After all, what did she and Wolf have in common, other than mutual attraction?

She didn't need all the window dressing. Just some good,

down-and-dirty sex. She hadn't even realized how much she missed it until a few days ago, when Wolf followed her out of the hotel and goaded her into joining him for lunch.

Just picturing him—that cocky grin, those dark brown eyes, the muscles that flexed with every move—brought back the same breathless, giddy feeling that pushed her to act so impulsively.

Hormones, that's all it was. And maybe some instinctive, fundamental need to connect with another human being on a purely physical level.

She wasn't looking for love. Not anymore. She'd buried that dream seven years ago, the same day they'd interred Nick's lifeless body in the ground.

But sex? That she could handle, in between her work commitments. No compromise of heart or mind required. Just a bed, some condoms, and a few hours of mutual pleasure.

Maybe she should have been more explicit when she called. Spelled out exactly what she wanted, instead of simply inviting him over after work on Friday.

"You cook?" Wolf said, voice raised over the sound of ringing phones, beeping telemetry monitors, someone calling for a nurse.

"No. Listen, if this isn't a good time, I can call back later—"

"Hang on, they're paging me." A brief exchange of muffled speech, and then he was back. "Sorry, it's been a zoo. Text me your address. You like Thai?"

"Yes, but—"

"Damn," he cut her off. In the background she could hear an overhead page that triggered memories of her own time in training: *Code blue, ICU. Code blue, ICU.* "Gotta go. See you Friday."

She vacillated over calling again the following day. But by the time she finished with meetings and conference calls, and waded through her inbox, her barely-there headache blossomed into a full-blown migraine that took her out of commission for the rest of Thursday and half of Friday. Which left her playing catch-up until after seven Friday night.

On the way home, an overturned tractor trailer snarled traffic for miles, and she had just enough time to shower and pull on some jeans and a tank top before the doorbell rang.

"Am I early?" Wolf said, taking in her wet hair and makeup-free face.

"No." She opened the door wider. "Come in."

The aroma of curry wafted up from the brown paper sack in his hand. Lily's stomach rumbled, reminding her that she hadn't eaten since noon.

Wolf followed her to the kitchen. "Where do you want this?"

"Counter's fine." She concentrated on setting the table, trying to keep her hands from trembling as he shed his leather jacket and draped it over a chair.

Stop staring. But it was hard to ignore the fluid movement of his body as he crossed to the kitchen sink to wash up. The way he filled out a pair of jeans…

Who was she kidding? There was no way she'd be able to keep her eyes off such temptation. The water cut off and she glanced up, flushing beneath his steady gaze.

"The hospital implemented this infection control campaign," he said, slowly drying his fingers on a paper towel. "There are signs everywhere. You know, like they have in restaurant bathrooms: *By California law, staff are required to wash their hands before returning to work.*"

She nodded and let out a breath. "Makes sense." Forcing herself to move, she retrieved the bag from the counter and started pulling out disposable containers.

"The problem is," he said, tossing out the paper towel, "every time I see one of those signs, it reminds me of an old joke."

"Which is…?"

"A doctor and a lawyer find themselves in the restroom at

the same time. The lawyer finishes, zips up, and heads for the door. The doctor stops him. 'You know,' he says, 'doctors always wash their hands after they urinate.' To which the lawyer replies, 'Yeah, but lawyers learn not to urinate on their hands!'"

She smiled. "You can use that as an ice-breaker at your next medical staff meeting."

"Yeah," he snorted. "Like the chief of staff doesn't hate me enough."

She raised a brow. "Why would he hate you?"

"Well, okay, maybe hate is too strong a word. Let's just say the guy doesn't get my sense of humor."

"Now *that* I can believe," she said. Especially since just last week, Wolf had aimed that barbed sense of humor in her direction. She didn't relish being anyone's target practice. And engaging Wolf in verbal sparring was like holding a lightning rod during an electric storm. Bad idea. Which was why she'd have preferred a booty call instead of dinner.

A shame he hadn't gotten the memo.

Though she had to admit that so far, he was being a model guest. Plus, she was hungry, and the food he'd brought smelled divine.

"Here." She handed him the Pad Thai. "Why don't you unload the rest while I get us something to drink? There's water, white wine—" she peered into the back of the fridge "—and beer."

"Beer's good, thanks."

She pulled out a dark bottle of Belgian ale left over from Parker's last visit and rummaged in the utensil drawer for a bottle opener.

"Can you do me a favor?" She pointed toward the pilsner glass on a top cabinet shelf. According to Parker, beer tasted better when drunk from proper glassware. "Can you get that for me?"

"This?" He reached up, his chest brushing her shoulder.

Her fingers jerked and she stilled, breathing in the scent of soap and cedar and the hint of something wild. Primal. Hot.

She ran her tongue over dry lips and tried to focus on the glass Wolf placed in front of her. When he reached for a second glass, she cleared her throat. "Just one. Thanks."

"You're not having any?"

"I don't really like beer." She opened the bottle and handed it over, then skirted past Wolf to fill a regular glass with ice and filtered tap water.

"Pretty fancy label for someone who doesn't like beer."

She waved him toward the table. "I have a friend who's a beer snob," she said as they filled their plates and sat down. "Goes to tastings and everything. You wouldn't believe the number of breweries there are between here and San Diego."

Wolf frowned. "Sounds like your friend and his liver should give the breweries a break."

She dipped a chicken satay skewer into the peanut sauce. "That's what I keep telling him."

"But he won't listen?"

"You ever try arguing with a lawyer?"

"Ah. Point taken," he said. "So does this beer-bellied friend live around here?"

She burst out laughing and nearly choked on a piece of chicken. Wolf shoved a glass of water in her hand and surged to his feet.

"I'm fine," she wheezed, waving him back down. "It's just that visual. Parker with a beer belly. Sorry…" She wiped her eyes with a napkin. "He ran the San Diego marathon in June. For the sixth time."

"Sixth time, huh?" He dug into the green curry. "Well, some people are slow learners. Maybe next time he'll get it right."

She grinned and shook her head. "Thanks. Really. I needed a good laugh."

"Glad to oblige," he said. "Tough week?"

"The usual." She took a sip of water, then set the glass down and resumed eating.

"Want to tell me about it?"

"Not really."

He blinked. "Why not?"

"Last time I tried, we got into an argument."

Wolf studied her for a long moment. "I'm not exactly your target audience."

"No. You're not." She smiled to soften the sting. "But you seem to be doing okay without my input."

"It's my patented humor-for-all-occasions approach."

"Whatever works."

For several minutes there was nothing but the scrape of cutlery on plates.

Wolf poured the rest of the beer into his glass. "Maybe you should try it."

"What, the beer?" Lily said. "Or cracking jokes?"

"The jokes, of course. See, you're already doing it. People respond to humor."

"There's a time and place. It's one thing if you're just hanging out, shooting the breeze. But I'm talking about serious issues."

"So? Nothing wrong with injecting a little humor, whatever the subject. Think of it as audience engagement."

She frowned.

"Here." He pushed aside his plate. "Let me show you something."

He pulled out his phone and dragged his chair closer. Turning the screen on its side, he tapped the familiar red and white icon and turned up the volume.

For a moment, she didn't register the action on-screen. The heat of Wolf's body, right next to her, was too distracting. His thigh brushed hers when he leaned in. His arm grazed her shoulders as he rested an elbow on the back of her chair.

And then the music filtered through and she did a double-take. The singer wore a police uniform complete with high black boots, hat, and reflective glasses. Behind him, a row of backup singers dressed as a biker, construction worker, soldier, cowboy, and tribal chieftain in feather headdress sang and danced across the stage to a familiar disco beat.

Young man, put your cigarette out.
I said, young man, 'cause there's really no doubt.
I said, young man, unless you want to fade out
While gasping hard for your last breath…

Lily glanced at Wolf, then back at the screen. "That's you?"

"Mm-hm. Keep watching."

Young man, you've heard that e-cigarettes,
Vaping, and hookahs are a way safer bet.
That's wrong, 'cause they're as much of a threat
To your lungs' viability.

The camera zoomed in on the backup singers, and Lily gasped. "No way—is that Doug Williams?"

"He prefers WildDogg MD," Wolf said. "At least when he's on camera."

"I can't believe it." She stared at the gyrating figures, each identical except for the costume. "I only met him once, but he seemed so…straight-laced."

"He is," Wolf laughed. "Most of the time."

Sing it with me now: C-O-P-D.
All together now: C-O-P-D.
That's what you get if you don't go smoke-free—
AKA em-phy-se-ma.

As the refrain repeated, Doug's characters dropped out one by one in a fit of coughing, until only Wolf remained standing. In the background, a second version of Wolf strutted onto the stage, dressed in scrubs and a stethoscope, and wheeling an oxygen tank and face mask.

The music faded. Credits rolled against a black backdrop. Wolf reappeared in scrubs, this time seated on a tall stool and illuminated by a single spotlight.

"COPD," he said, addressing the camera directly, "or chronic obstructive pulmonary disease, is the third leading cause of death in the U.S. Sixteen million Americans struggle with the condition every day. Typical symptoms include shortness of breath—"

Wolf tapped the screen, but Lily grabbed his wrist before he could press pause. "Wait, I want to see."

The remaining forty-five seconds covered the basics: symptoms, treatment, prevention, and concluded with Wolf's impassioned plea against the top cause of the disease, smoking.

"Wow." Lily looked up at him. "That was amazing. You and Doug did it all yourselves?"

"Mostly." He glanced at her fingers, still resting atop his wrist. She flushed and pulled away. Lips quirking, he turned off the phone. "We hired a cameraman, sound engineer, and someone to do the lighting. But the rest...yeah."

"Do you have more videos?"

"Close to a hundred at last count."

Her brows shot up. "A *hundred?* All with medical themes?"

"Pretty much."

"Wow," she said again. If she hadn't just watched the video herself, she would never have believed it. "Can I see some of the others?"

"You can look them up yourself. Just Google 'Wolfman MD.' You can even subscribe to our YouTube channel." He set aside the phone. "So, anyway, do you see what I mean about using humor, even when dealing with something that's not inherently funny?"

"I guess." She picked up her fork again. "Though I still think some topics should be off limits. Like depression and suicide. You just don't joke about things like that."

"Why not?"

His question dumbfounded her. "I would think that's obvious. You don't exploit someone's personal tragedy for the sake of a cheap laugh."

"It's not exploitation if the purpose is to raise awareness," he countered. "Particularly if it's a topic that would otherwise be overlooked or dismissed."

Okay, maybe he had a point. *If* the topic were anything

other than the one under discussion. But the consequences of mental illness were no laughing matter.

"So," she said, "you're telling me that you would make a music video about physician suicide?"

"*I* wouldn't," he said. "Too much of a downer. But if you're so interested in the topic, maybe *you* should."

"Oh, sure. I'll pencil it in for the twelfth of never."

He laughed and shook his head. "You are one incredibly stubborn woman."

"I prefer the term *principled.*"

"Yeah, I guess you would." He leaned back in his chair and watched her eat.

Self-conscious under the close scrutiny, Lily turned the conversation back to him. "How'd you get into doing music videos?"

"Luck. Or fate. Maybe a little of both." He finished off his beer. "You know how you get a song stuck in your head? Maybe a catchy tune, or some syncopated rhythm, and you just can't get rid of it? As a kid, I'd play around with the lyrics. And then I heard Weird Al Yankovic and it was like a light bulb went off. By the time I got to med school, I was primed. I'd get together with friends to jam, and we'd pick a song and make up our own lyrics. And when you hang out with med students, the conversation inevitably revolves around shit that happens on rounds, or in the O.R., or whatever rotation you're on."

"So you've been doing this since med school?"

"More or less. We didn't start recording and posting videos online until a few years ago."

Lily glanced at his empty glass. "Another beer?"

"No, thanks." He pushed back his chair. "But I'll get some water. You want a refill?"

"I can—"

"No, I'll get it. You eat." He rose and reached across for her glass.

She nearly dropped her fork when his hip brushed against her, but managed to recover her composure by the time he returned with the water. "Thanks."

He resumed his seat, putting a bit more distance between them.

She tamped down her disappointment and speared a few green beans. "Did you study singing?"

"Nah, I'm a natural." He grinned. "But I did take piano lessons. We all did. My mom's a piano teacher, so I guess it comes with the territory."

"And by 'all' you mean…"

"My brothers and I."

She cocked her head. "How many brothers do you have?"

"Three."

"There are *three more* like you?"

"Hell, no. I'm better looking and way smarter than those jokers."

She blinked, then narrowed her eyes. "More arrogant, maybe."

"I'm hurt," he said. "You haven't even met my brothers, and you're already taking their side."

"No, just calling it as I see it," she said. "What about your father? Is he a musician too?"

"No. Dad had a tin ear. But he appreciated our efforts. He taught history and coached high school football."

"Is he retired?"

"No. He died at forty. Pancreatic cancer."

"Oh, no. I'm so sorry."

He nodded and looked around, as if searching for something else to focus on. "You have siblings?"

"No." She reached for her water and took a sip. "How'd you go from playing piano as a kid to doing musical parodies now?"

He shrugged. "I grew up wanting to do hip-hop."

Her brows shot up.

"Yeah, I know," he said. "That was me, rebelling. When your mom worships at the altar of Johann Sebastien Bach, and names all her children after classical composers—"

"You're kidding."

"Swear to God. Sebastien—" he ticked the names off on his fingers "—after J.S. Bach, of course. He got the crap kicked out of him at school until he shortened it to Seb and learned to fight back. Then yours truly, after Wolfgang Amadeus Mozart. And if you repeat that, I will haunt you to your dying day."

She mimed the zipping of her lips. "Not a word."

He nodded. "That brings us to the twins. Since they came last, they got stuck with the less important composers. Georg Friedrich Handel and Franz Joseph Haydn."

"Dare I ask…?"

"Freddy and Joe," he said. "Nice, normal names, except when they have to show a driver's license or passport."

"I can see why classical music was a nonstarter. What happened to hip-hop?"

"Reality intruded." He sighed. "Dad got sick. Six months later, he was gone. Money, which was tight to begin with, got even tighter. So I stopped trying to be a rebel. Figured there was more financial security in medicine, anyway."

"You don't regret it?"

"Giving up hip-hop? Nah. I wasn't that good anyway. At least not good enough to make a career out of it."

"What about medicine? Any regrets there?"

He shook his head. "I like taking care of patients. Most of the time. And as a hospitalist, I average seven days on, seven days off. Plenty of time to play around with music and have fun. Frankly, if I had to choose just one—medicine or music—I think I'd be bored. This way, I get to enjoy the best of both worlds."

Lily studied him. "So it all worked out."

"Yes," he said. "It did. What about you?"

"What about me?" She got up and started clearing the table.

Wolf rose to help. "Are you happy with this whole lecture circuit/motivational speaking thing?"

She paused. "You mean my advocacy work."

"Yeah, that."

She gritted her teeth and resumed cleaning. Was he even aware of how insulting that sounded? The easy rapport they'd built over dinner dissipated, like a layer of mist burned off by the sun, leaving behind a harsh landscape she had no interest in navigating.

Tossing the empty containers in the trash, she crossed to the sink, where Wolf was stacking dirty dishes.

"I'll take care of this," she said, reaching for the dish-washing fluid. "Thanks for bringing dinner."

He ceded his spot at the sink, but remained close enough for her to feel his presence beside her.

Hip propped against the counter, he watched as she attacked the plates with a scrub sponge. "Are you kicking me out?"

She hesitated. "No. I just don't feel like arguing."

"Good. Neither do I."

"It's just…" She bit her lip.

"Just what?"

She shook her head and rinsed off each plate, then loaded the dishwasher.

"Lily." He stepped closer and shut off the faucet.

She glared up at him. "You're giving me whiplash."

"Excuse me?"

"Being all nice and funny and then—bam!—reverting to Mr. Neanderthal."

His lips twitched and he took another step, crowding her against the edge of the sink. Leaning in, he planted his hands on the counter on either side of her. "If you're going to call me names, at least get the title right. That's *Dr.* Neanderthal, thank you very much."

His proximity was making it hard to breathe. Hard to think. She pressed back against the hard surface behind her. "You think this is funny?"

"Help me out here." His lips grazed her ear. "What are you really mad about?"

She pressed her wet hands against his chest. Beneath the soft cotton of his shirt, she could feel the rapid staccato of his heart. "You're treating what I do as a joke."

"I asked if you're happy with your work." The rasp of his

day-old beard against her cheek made her shiver. "I'm sorry if you found that offensive."

"It's the *way* you said it."

"The *way*...?" He lifted his head, staring down at her. "Is this one of those twists of logic that anyone with a Y chromosome has no hope of following?"

She reared back, eyes flaring. "See, you're doing it again."

"Doing *what* again?"

"Acting like a condescending, sexist jerk."

The arms around her loosened. He stepped back and sighed. "Look, it's clear we both had a rough week. So how about we cut each other some slack? Pretend like the last ten minutes didn't happen."

"Just like that," she said, crossing her arms over her chest. "No apologies, just click rewind and all is forgiven."

"Yeah, I can see that's not happening." He rubbed a hand over the back of his neck. "I think I'd better go."

She lifted her chin. "Yes. Maybe you should."

For several seconds, neither of them moved.

Then he nodded and turned away. She watched him retrieve his phone from the table and don the leather jacket.

That was it? He was just going to leave?

After priming her with funny stories...

And teasing her with tantalizing glimpses of the man behind the pretty face...

And ratcheting up the sexual tension to the point where she was almost ready to say the hell with it, and jump his bones...

After all that, he was leaving?

"Wait," she said.

He halted, halfway to the door. Glanced back. "Yes?"

"I wanted to say...thank you. For dinner. And for coming over." She trailed off and bit her lip. The silence lengthened.

His eyes searched her face, looking for...what?

She gripped the edge of the sink behind her. "It was very nice of you."

"I don't do nice," he said. And then he headed for the door. "Goodnight, Lily."

The snick of the automatic lock echoed in the empty hall. Lily closed her eyes and sagged against the counter. "Idiot." She wasn't sure if she meant Wolf or herself.

CHAPTER FOUR

Despite feeling exhausted, she couldn't sleep.

She tried her usual go-to remedies. Warm milk, deep breathing, reading technical papers until her eyes glazed over. Nothing helped.

The problem was her thoughts kept drifting back to Wolf.

The evening she'd anticipated hadn't materialized. Instead, he'd thrown her off balance from the moment he stepped over the threshold and swept aside her plans for seduction. Granted, she hadn't tried too hard nor objected too much when food and conversation took center stage. But somewhere between the chicken satay appetizer and the kiss that never happened, he'd managed to win her over. And then alienate her again. All in the space of a few hours.

Having a dinner that started with such promise end in disappointment left her more physically frustrated than she'd been in years.

Finally giving up on sleep, she pulled out her iPad.

A few mind-numbing rounds of solitaire later, she opened a browser window and typed in *Wolfman MD*. In under a second, Google spit out two hundred thousand hits.

She scrolled quickly through the first few pages. Interviews and guest appearances on dozens of medical news sites, blogs, and digital editions of newspapers. *USA Today*, the *L.A. Times*, *The Wall Street Journal*. There was even a brief entry in Wikipedia that dubbed him "the dopest medical satirist and cross-genre musician in healthcare today."

From there, a link took her to YouTube, where she spent the next couple hours binge-watching his videos. Doug appeared in many of them, and a few included other people in bit roles as well. The humor ranged from witty to downright crass. But whatever he was doing, it seemed to be working: some of the videos had garnered over ten million views, and none had fewer than ten thousand. Something about Wolfman & WildDogg, or MD^2, as the duo billed themselves, attracted a devoted following. Their YouTube channel boasted eight million subscribers. *Eight million.*

If Lily could appeal to one tenth that number—or even a hundredth—she'd be thrilled.

The Kickstarter campaign she launched last year to crowdfund a documentary about physician suicide expired long before it got even halfway toward goal. Since then, she'd relegated the project to the back burner. She still mentioned it in passing at workshops or during media appearances, hoping to attract enough attention and maybe some corporate sponsorship to resuscitate it. The one-page synopsis she'd mentioned to Wolf last week was ready and waiting for anyone who expressed an interest.

But the reality was, no one wanted to hear the truth. It remained medicine's dirty little secret that doctors, charged with treating the ill and vulnerable, were themselves suffering and even dying from the unrelenting stress of an often toxic work environment.

Only those physicians directly affected by it—and possibly their closest family and friends—dared acknowledge the silent epidemic. For the rest, depression and suicide remained a taboo subject. Admitting to feeling depressed still carried tremendous stigma in the medical community, and had the potential to derail a physician's career.

So while Lily touched on the subject, she tended to talk

more about burnout—a politically correct, more palatable term for what ailed so many physicians.

Thinking about the many orders of magnitude that separated her under-represented audience from the massive fan base enjoyed by Wolf, she felt a fresh wave of resentment and despair.

If vulgar humor was what attracted fans, she might as well hang up her microphone now, because she refused to go there. Wolf might have no problem dropping f-bombs, but for her to adopt that approach would be demeaning. An insult to the dead whose memory she'd pledged to honor, and to the living whose pain she was trying to heal.

She shut down her iPad and stared at the ceiling. It was nearly four in the morning when she finally managed to fall asleep.

"You look wiped out," Parker said later, as they sat at an outside table and waited for their meal.

On less than five hours' sleep, she wasn't surprised. Ordinarily she'd have covered the dark under-eye smudges with makeup. But she'd been running late all morning, and it was a two-and-a-half hour drive to Encinitas. Besides, this was Parker. He'd seen her in much worse condition than this.

She shrugged off his concern. "You know how it is. Work, travel. The usual."

"What you need is a vacation," he said. "When's the last time you took any time off? I bet you can't even remember."

He was right, but she wasn't about to admit it. "Did you bring the Wiggs file?"

"Yes," he sighed. "But can we eat first? I skipped breakfast."

Right on cue, the waitress brought out their orders.

Lily eyed the monstrosity on Parker's plate. "That looks like breakfast, lunch, and dinner combined."

"It's called efficiency," he said, liberally dousing the multilayered burger with ketchup and hot sauce. "Sure you don't want one of these babies yourself?"

"Positive." She sprinkled walnuts and raisins on her oatmeal. "Not everyone is lucky enough to have your metabolism."

"Darlin', luck has nothin' to do with it. Takes hard work to look this good. And you—" he eyed her figure, or at least what was visible above the table "—have nothin' to worry about."

"Thanks," she said dryly.

He grinned and dove into the burger. "So you want to tell me what's really botherin' you?"

The oatmeal turned to wet cardboard in her mouth. After a few spoonfuls, she gave up. "You think what we're doing here will make any difference?"

He didn't even hesitate. "To Sara Wiggs it will."

"True," Lily sighed. "But even if she wins the case, and the residency program agrees to take her back and pay damages, they're not going to admit that what happened to her is a systemic problem."

"These things take time," he said. "You need to have patience."

"I do. But it's frustrating."

"Trust me, I know." He took another bite and studied her as he chewed. "This isn't the first case we've taken on, and it won't be the last. We've planted the seed for change, and every judgment in our favor helps it grow."

"Is that another one of your down-home aphorisms?"

"Nope. That one's all me. Feel free to use it."

She cradled her coffee mug in both hands. "Do you think this'll go to trial?"

"Probably not. If our arguments are convincin' enough, it'll be cheaper and less of a PR nightmare for the hospital to settle out of court."

"Not much of a sacrifice for them," Lily said. "Quiet settlement for some undisclosed amount, no admission of guilt, and they'll probably insist that Sara sign a non-disclosure agreement to keep her from going public."

"Yes, but at least she'll get her spot back, provided she still wants it. And I'll make sure she gets compensatory as well as punitive damages. Not a bad outcome, if you ask me."

"I guess."

"Lily." Parker furrowed his brow. "This case is about Sara, not about you or me or anyone else. It may not fix the system, but it's a step in the right direction."

Lily finished her coffee. "You're right. Of course you're right."

"And if they don't settle," he said, "or if they try to drag things out, we'll go to the media. Start makin' the rounds. Everyone loves a human interest story. Sara's young, she's pretty, she's got cancer. The public will lap it up. Young doctor-in-trainin' falls ill, and her residency program embarks on a passive-aggressive campaign that makes it impossible for her to get treatment and still keep her job. Discrimination, intimidation, retaliation. It's all there."

"Like a Greek tragedy."

"Except with a happier endin'," he said. "And in order to get there, I need your help siftin' through the latest depositions. All that medical jargon."

"Coming from a lawyer—"

"Yeah, yeah, we all have our crosses to bear." He wiped his hands and mouth with a napkin. "Bottom line, the residency program violated federal statutes. Doctors aren't exempt from protection under the Americans with Disabilities Act or Family Medical Leave Act. I'm fixin' to drive that point home, and y'all will help me. Whatever it takes, we will prevail. In court, out of court, in the court of public opinion. Okay?"

She took a deep breath and nodded. "Thanks."

"Don't mention it. We're in this together, Lil. You just keep bringin' me the cases."

"You don't have enough pro bono work?"

"I'm serious. If we do it enough times, med schools and residency programs will start takin' notice. They won't have a choice."

She reached across the table to squeeze his hand. "Thank

you."

"Anytime." His fingers tightened around hers. "Lily…"

"Yes?"

His pale gray eyes focused on her face. For a moment he didn't say anything. Then he opened his mouth and—

"How are you folks doing?" their waitress interrupted. "Anything more I can get you?"

Parker sighed and let go. "Some coffee," he said. "And more creamer. Lil?"

"Water, please."

"Sure thing," the woman said. "And if you're done with this, I can take your plates."

They waited in silence while she cleared the table.

Once they were alone again, Lily glanced at Parker. "You were about to say something."

He hesitated, then shook his head. "Nothin' important. You ready to get to work?"

For the next hour, over several refills of coffee, they pored over documents while Parker took notes on his laptop.

"That should do it," he finally said, shutting down the computer and packing everything away. "I'll write it up and send you the draft for review by Monday. You have plans for the rest of the weekend?"

She rose and winced as stiff muscles protested. "Just catching up on everything I didn't do last week."

"Well, now," he said. "I have a better idea. Why don't you stay a couple days, take a break? It's a long drive back. And work'll still be there next week."

"I can't," Lily said. "But I wouldn't turn down a walk before I head out."

After a brief detour to pay the bill and use the restroom, they set off at a leisurely pace to explore the neighborhood.

"You know what really burns me?" Lily said.

"What?"

"Here we are, working so hard to do good, and we're barely moving the needle. I mean, sure, we're helping a few people like Sara. And maybe I'm reaching some of the docs who attend my workshops or hear me talk. But we're dealing with an epidemic here. If people just realized how important and pervasive the problem is, they'd be lining up in droves to support a documentary that spreads the word."

"Maybe Kickstarter just wasn't the right platform."

"It's not like I was asking for the moon. In today's world, five hundred thousand for a full-length documentary is a bargain. And with crowdfunding, a person could contribute any amount. Whatever they were comfortable with. Five dollars. Ten. Anything. People stop by Starbucks on the way to work every day and spend more on a coffee and bagel. I mean, come on, am I being unreasonable?"

"Not at all. And my offer's still good—"

"I know, Parker." She wrapped an arm around his. "And I love you for it. But I won't let you risk your life savings on something that's probably going to lose money."

"It's not exactly my life savin's," he said. "And I can always earn it back. That's the beauty of billable hours. Especially when you have a law school buddy who happens to be in-house counsel at San Diego's biggest marketing agency and is always willin' to throw you extra work."

Ah. Parker's mysterious "buddy," without whom an outsider from North Carolina like Parker would never have made it in San Diego's insular legal community.

Lily suspected the man did more than just funnel work Parker's way. But Parker never discussed his sex life with her, and she never asked. None of her business, anyway.

Money, on the other hand, was a different story. And she could not, in good conscience, allow Parker to finance her project. He wasn't a trust fund baby, the way Nick had been.

"It's too much," she said. "You're already doing all this pro bono and contingency work—"

"He was my best friend, Lil."

She bit her lip and nodded. "I know."

For several minutes, they walked in silence. Off the main drag, the streets were narrow, lined with modest houses and minuscule yards. A dog barked somewhere in the distance.

"What about your daddy?" Parker said.

She sighed. "He's still mad that I dropped out of residency. According to him, I'm wasting my life, and until I give up this nonsense there's nothing to talk about."

"Son of a—" he broke off. "That man's got more dollars than sense. You're not givin' up, are you?"

"Of course not. But I may need to rethink my approach." She chewed her lip. "Lighten up a little. Maybe use humor as a hook."

"Humor," Parker repeated, as if he'd never heard the word. "When talkin' about suicide."

"Not suicide. But maybe burnout…" She faltered. "What's that line…Ten million fans can't be wrong?"

"It's fifty million Elvis fans can't be wrong. And this is apropos of…?"

"If someone has a fan base of millions, they've got to be doing something right."

"Depends. You got someone particular in mind, or we still talkin' hypotheticals?"

"Well, this guy Wolf—"

"Wait a minute." Parker frowned and slowed to a stop, forcing Lily to stop as well. "This the guy you had lunch with last week?"

"Yes."

"The one you told me to report to the police if I didn't hear from you within two hours?"

"Well…yes. But I *did* call you back in less than two hours—"

"After I nearly had a heart attack because you turned off your phone and I couldn't reach you."

"Come on, Parker," Lily said. "I already apologized for that."

"Fine. Just don't you ever scare me like that again."

"I won't." She tugged on his arm, and they resumed walking. "Can we get back to the subject?"

"Fine."

"So, anyway, Wolf has this side gig. Takes popular songs

and writes his own lyrics and then makes parody videos. He and his friend Doug—they go by Wolfman and WildDogg MD—have built a huge following. We're talking millions of people watching these videos." She paused as Parker's frown deepened. "I'll admit, some of it's way over the top. But a lot of the videos are funny. And spot on. They'd have to be. I mean, they're both doctors, and the videos deal with all sorts of medical issues—"

"Hold on," Parker said. "What are their names again?"

"Wolfman and WildDogg. They call themselves MD^2."

"No, I mean their real names."

"Wolf Knox and Doug Williams. Why?"

"Doug Williams. Of course. That's why this was startin' to sound familiar."

"What are you talking about?"

"There was a lawsuit. Two, three years ago. Some celebrity sued a couple physicians for defamation of character. I remember readin' about it. Sounded plumb crazy."

"Why?"

"Because Doug Williams is the last person you'd expect to be involved in somethin' like that. I went to school with him, pledged the same fraternity. He was always quiet. Super smart, but not the kind to make waves."

"Small world." Lily said. "How'd the lawsuit turn out?"

"Beats me." He shrugged. "I had other things to worry about, so it just fell off my radar. If you're curious, I'm sure we could find out."

"Yes, let's. You can call Doug—"

"I meant we could look up the information online."

Lily wrinkled her nose. "Wouldn't it be easier to just pick up the phone?"

He narrowed his eyes. "Okay, Lil, out with it. What are you really after?"

"Millions of viewers. Can you imagine if we had that kind of reach?"

"You want access to their viewers."

"Yes. Wouldn't it be amazing? They could do a video for

us. Obviously, with strict oversight of the content, to make sure it's appropriate…or at least not offensive. Wolf does these little public service announcements at the end of each video, on whatever the topic is. All in plain English. If he did one about depression or burnout among physicians—"

Parker cut her off before she could get too carried away. "Did y'all talk to him about it?"

"In passing."

"And…?"

Her eyes slid away from Parker's. "He said no."

"In other words, it doesn't matter how big their fan base is. If they already refused—"

"*Wolf* refused. But maybe Doug would agree. I mean, he's obviously got some vested interest in the topic. He chairs the Physician Health Committee at Saint Mary's. He was the one who reached out to me about doing last week's talk. Why wouldn't he agree to something like this? And if he agrees, maybe he can talk Wolf into doing it too."

Parker shook his head. "You're barkin' up the wrong tree."

"I'm thinking outside the box."

"Fine, then. Here. Use my phone." He fished it out. "Go ahead, call him."

She pushed his hand away. "I can't go behind Wolf's back. But *you* could call your friend Doug, and just not mention me…"

"*Friend* is a gross exaggeration. He was three years ahead, a senior by the time Nick and I rushed…" Parker trailed off. "I haven't seen the guy in years."

"Please. If not for me, then for Nick."

His lips tightened. "You're not playin' fair, Lil."

The familiar rush of guilt made it hard to swallow. "I'm sorry. Forget I said anything."

Parker nodded and they continued down the street in silence.

Several blocks later, he sighed. "Fine, you win. I'll do it."

"You'll call?"

"Yes. But before y'all get too excited, realize that this is a long shot. The guy might not even remember me."

"Thank you." She threw her arms around him. "You're the best."

"Yeah," Parker said. "That's what they tell me."

She closed her eyes. Her thoughts drifted back to last night, and a different pair of arms.

How would Wolf react when he discovered what she'd done?

An unexpected surge of excitement quickened her pulse.

Later, she'd try to rationalize it. Bury her guilt beneath layers of altruistic intent.

But for now, she acknowledged the shameful truth. Her excitement had nothing to do with the video she wanted Wolf to make—and everything to do with the man himself.

CHAPTER FIVE

Wolf had never been keen on kids. They were loud, expensive, messy, and they took over your entire life.

Buh-bye, sleep. Buh-bye, privacy. Buh-bye, sex.

All excellent reasons for leaving the task of procreation to his brothers, who had no such qualms about producing bumper crops of mini-mes. They did so regularly enough that Wolf had more nieces and nephews than he could count.

And now Doug—who'd been happy playing Wolf's wingman since med school—had broken ranks. Husband and father, all within a year. Fuck. Maybe there was something in the water.

Wolf sat on the living room couch and watched Doug pace, screaming child cradled against his chest. Amid the explosion of baby paraphernalia, this seemed the safest place to sit and drink one of the beers he'd brought over. The food remained on the kitchen table, untouched. It should probably be put in the fridge, unless Doug managed to calm the kid down in the next ten minutes.

"Maybe he's hungry," Wolf said, wincing as the cries became more strident. He was surprised that Tina hadn't popped out to see what the caterwauling was all about. Then again, she was barely ten days out from an emergency Csection, and probably so frazzled and sleep deprived from breastfeeding and dealing with a newborn that it was no wonder she'd handed off her son and holed up in the bedroom the moment Wolf arrived.

"He can't be hungry." Doug adjusted his hold and continued walking a path across the carpet. "Tina just fed him. I burped him and changed his diaper, so that's not it. No fever. Belly's soft. He's probably just tired."

"Last I checked," Wolf said, "the cure for that was sleep. That sound like sleep to you?"

Doug sighed. "I guess I could try swaddling him."

Miraculously, the crying stopped. Within minutes, the baby was asleep in a bassinet in the corner. Doug sank down on an armchair nearby and rested his head against the cushioned back.

"You look like you could use a beer," Wolf said.

"Too tired to get up."

Wolf set his half-finished bottle down and headed for the kitchen, bringing back the rest of the six-pack and a bottle opener. He popped the cap off a bottle. "Here."

"Thanks." They sat for several minutes in blessed silence.

Wolf lounged back and propped his feet up on the coffee table, glad Tina wasn't there to see it. "There's food."

"Later." Doug took another long pull on the bottle. "I had an interesting call the other day. A fellow UCSD alum. Parker Atkinson."

Parker? Wolf frowned. Not the most common of names. And he'd heard it recently. Probably just a coincidence.

"He's a lawyer now," Doug continued. "Does some litigation on behalf of physicians."

Okay, maybe not a coincidence. Wolf's frown deepened. "What did he want?"

"Said he'd seen some of our work and has an idea for a new video."

"Oh, yeah?" Wolf said. "What about?"

Not that he had any intention of taking Parker the lawyer's suggestion, but he was curious. It wasn't unusual for fans to email or comment on their videos. And they all had ideas for the Funniest Video Ever.

Doug hesitated. "Physician burnout—"

"No," Wolf snapped, then glanced toward the corner. Through the sheer mesh sides of the bassinet, he could see the baby sleeping. He lowered his voice. "Absolutely not. And I hope you told him that."

"Well…not exactly."

"Which part of *'hell, no'* did you not get?"

Doug leaned forward. "Remember Pink Floyd? *The Wall?*"

"What about it?"

"There's this scene where an endless line of kids shuffles toward a conveyor belt that feeds them into a giant meat grinder. It's perfect. I can totally picture it. Zombies in white coats lining up—"

"Forget it."

"At least hear me out," Doug said. "I've been playing around with the lyrics."

He stood up and patted his pockets, then looked around until he spotted a cell phone sticking out from an outside pocket of a diaper bag. Device in hand, he perched on the edge of the sofa beside Wolf and cued a sound track. "Listen to this…"

Despite himself, Wolf did. The tinny music, with haunting lyrics sung in a monotone, sent shivers up his spine. It was a relief when Doug turned down the volume, but the reprieve didn't last long. Doug hummed a few bars, then started singing softly, layering his own words over the original.

We don't need your innovation.
We don't need your brain at all.
We just need your blind allegiance
To our corporate protocol.
Hey! Doctor! Your work's not done yet.
See more patients, check more boxes, write prescriptions.
Stick to treating only authorized conditions.

We don't care if you're exhausted.
We don't care if you are sick.
You have not fulfilled your quota.
Do we need a bigger stick?
Hey! Doctor! Your work's not done yet...

Doug's voice trailed off. "It's rough, I know. But you get the idea."

Wolf shook his head, annoyed at himself for even considering it. "Count me out."

"That's it?" Doug glared at him. "Just *'count me out*'?"

"What did you expect me to say? *'Nice job, let's do it*'?"

"Maybe not, but I hoped…" Doug tossed the phone onto the coffee table and crossed the room to the bassinet. For several minutes he stood there, watching his son sleep. Then he sighed and returned to the armchair. "I've been thinking about this a while, even before Parker's call. Having a kid changes things. I want more balance in my life. More family time. I want to see my son grow up. Surely you, of all people, can understand that."

Wolf scowled. "My father *died*. Which, in case you missed that day in med school, is a permanent, irreversible state. What you're talking about is totally different. You work, you come home. You're still there for your son."

"Okay," Doug said. "You're right. It's not the same thing. But there are only so many hours in a day, and I don't want to spend them all working."

Wolf shook his head. "You're going soft, bro."

"No. I'm learning to prioritize." He reached for his beer again. "Let me put it this way. At the end of the day, what would you regret more: not working enough, or not spending enough time with your wife and kid?"

"I don't have a wife and kid."

"If you did…"

"Just because you drank the Kool-Aid doesn't mean I plan to," Wolf said. "Not everyone's looking to settle for a life of domestic bliss."

"And here I was, hoping the Postgraduate Assembly might have changed your mind."

Wolf narrowed his eyes. "Why would you think that?"

"Just a rumor. Something about you leaving with the keynote speaker."

"Ah, that. Didn't work out."

"Too bad."

Wolf shrugged. "She wasn't my type anyway."

He ignored Doug's disbelieving look. So what if he still got hard just thinking about Lily? Who could blame him? In jeans and tank top, or fully made up and wrapped in that sexy librarian outfit—it didn't matter. The woman was seriously hot.

But she also had a chip the size of Texas on her shoulder. And some crazy-ass notions that might apply in some fantasy world but were completely impractical in real life.

It was all well and good to talk about work-life balance, but the truth was it didn't exist. Not in medicine. Or at least not in the sense Doug was nattering on about. Balance in the real world was having someone in the background, taking care of all the details that made the day run smoothly. It was delegating the childcare, cooking, cleaning, laundry, shopping, errands, and whatever else took your attention away from work. Sure, there were some part-timers out there who claimed they could do it all. But man, what a waste of an education. That was like asking the CEO of Morgan Stanley to balance your checkbook. Sure he could do it, but his skills were better put to use overseeing billion dollar transactions.

Whatever bug had crawled up Doug's ass, he'd be back to his usual self once he returned to work. They'd been through med school and residency together, and that was before Doug signed on for an additional three years of fellowship training in pulmonary and critical care medicine. The man knew how to work hard. Having a kid, no matter what he said now, wasn't going to change that.

As for Lily, she simply didn't get it. Wolf had tried to explain it to her, that first day over lunch. Being a doctor was like going off to war as part of an elite military force. It was a test of character and endurance, and only the strong survived. That's why the training had to be so rigorous, and anyone who complained or dropped out wasn't fit for duty anyway.

Sure, not everyone shared his views. Wolf didn't mind a difference of opinion. What drove him nuts was people who wouldn't shut up about it, who insisted on ramming their beliefs down your throat, and then got all bent out of shape when you dared to argue.

He had enough crap to deal with at work. He didn't want to deal with it in his personal life too. Eventually, his dick would get the message. Then he'd be able to move on to a more restful woman who put her mouth to better use than going on and on about a subject he considered closed.

Later, on the drive home, Wolf found himself humming the tune from *The Wall*.

Cursing, he turned on the radio.

Beethoven's *Ode to Joy*. Brilliant.

He turned it up to full blast, drowning out the noise in his head.

In the end, he couldn't drown it out completely.

Not when Lily kept popping into his thoughts at random times.

It was his week off, so he didn't have work to distract him. And every time he sat down at the keyboard or picked up his headphones, he kept hearing that damn song Doug planted in his head.

Frustrated, he grabbed his board and drove up to Malibu. It was unseasonably cold for mid-October, and aside from Wolf and a few locals in wetsuits, the beach was nearly deserted.

As he paddled out to the lineup, the initial shock of hitting icy water dissipated, and he could feel himself entering the zone. For the first hour, he rode an adrenaline high. A stiff crosswind made for choppy waters—which under normal circumstances, would have posed no problem.

But then his eyes locked on a couple he hadn't noticed before. They were walking along the shoreline, holding hands. Something about the woman reminded him of Lily. And that was all it took to blow his concentration.

He managed to catch a wave, but wiped out two seconds later. Water closed over his head, and for a moment he was too disoriented from being rag-dolled to know which way was up. Then survival instinct kicked in, and he swam toward the light, desperate to reach the surface before his air ran out.

Back on shore, he released the Velcro strap of his leash, which had miraculously stayed attached, stuck his board in the sand, and collapsed beside it, still breathing hard.

"Dude, you okay?"

Wolf opened his eyes and squinted at the silhouette looming over him. It took a few seconds to recognize the male half of the couple he'd seen earlier.

The woman stood several feet away. At this distance, Wolf could tell that she was older than Lily, with thinner lips and the wrong color eyes, and the perpetually startled expression of someone who'd had one too many plastic surgeries.

"He looks fine," she said, tugging on her companion's arm. "Let's go."

Wolf dredged up a smile, which seemed to reassure the man enough to offer sympathy over the gnarly waves before moving on.

The following day, Wolf loaded up his mountain bike and headed for Will Rogers Park.

Halfway through the fourteen mile loop of the Backbone Trail, he started wondering what Lily did for fun. She talked about the importance of extracurricular activities to reduce stress, but failed to mention which specific ones she enjoyed. Come to think of it, she didn't talk much about herself at all. Her work, yes. She could hold forth ad nauseum about that. But when it came to answering personal questions, she had an uncanny knack for changing the subject. Which both intrigued and frustrated him.

It also left plenty of room for speculation. And speculate he did.

She probably did yoga. He could easily picture her in Lycra, her supple body bending, stretching, each sinuous move choreographed for seduction.

His fingers tightened on the handlebars, and he imagined touching her, running his hands down the smooth column of her spine, curving around that slender waist, grasping those rounded hips, bending her forward until that heart-shaped ass pressed back against his groin. He could almost feel the heat of her as he slid one hand forward, parting her thighs—

And that was when his bike skidded off the trail and into the dense underbrush that broke his fall. He lay there for a minute, stunned. Then he hauled himself up and rescued his bike, inspecting it for damage. A few dings, but otherwise remarkably intact. He brushed off the bits of foliage and dirt that clung to him, cleaned the worst of his scrapes with bottled water, and readjusted his helmet for the ride back.

He really needed to get his shit together. Stop fantasizing about a woman who was not only bad for his ego, but actually proving dangerous to his health.

His determination lasted all the way home. It melted a little in the steamy confines of his shower, and evaporated completely when the phone rang and Lily's voice reached out across the wireless connection like a physical force, stroking his libido.

"Do you have some free time this week?" she said. "I still owe you dinner."

"No—" he cleared his throat. "I mean, you don't owe me anything."

"Okay. I'd *like* to buy you dinner. Unless that was a polite brush-off, and you really don't want to see me. I'm a little rusty at this dating thing. I'm not sure it's even called that anymore. I keep hearing about this hookup culture—"

"When?" he said, cutting her off before she managed to talk them both out of it.

"Tomorrow? Seven? Or if you're busy—"

"Where?"

"There are some great restaurants on Lincoln, just south of the Marina. And on Pacific Avenue, if you want something closer to the water. Or…" she hesitated, and in that infinitesimal pause, he understood how Odysseus felt, tied to the mast of his ship as it sailed past the Sirens. "We could eat in. At my place."

"Your place it is," he said. Tomorrow night at seven. Jesus, he hoped he could last until then. "What should I bring?"

"Nothing. I'll order in. Is there anything you don't eat?"

"Monkey brains."

Her ripple of laughter brought an answering smile to his lips. "No monkey brains. Got it."

He hung up, still smiling.

Now if he could just avoid any further mishaps before tomorrow night….

He showed up at seven on the dot, with a bottle of wine and a box of chocolates.

"Mm, you smell good," he said, leaning in and taking an exaggerated whiff.

Lily stepped back, and for a moment he got the same sinking feeling he remembered from childhood, whenever he overdid it with the wisecracks and got sent to the principal's office.

Then Lily fluttered her lashes and smiled. "It's my new perfume. *Eau de souvlaki.*"

Wolf grinned. Maybe the evening wouldn't end in disaster after all.

He followed her to the kitchen, drinking in the sight of her sexy-as-fuck body poured into skinny black jeans and lacy white top. Her hair was up in a casual twist that looked like it could come tumbling down any second. His fingers itched to speed the process.

She turned, catching him mid-ogle. But instead of giving

him the evil eye, like she had the first time they'd met, she caught his gaze and then did a slow once-over that had him standing at attention in jeans that were suddenly a couple sizes too tight.

"Make yourself at home." She nodded toward the sink. "There's also a restroom down the hall that way."

"Thanks," he said. "I'll be right back."

It took a few minutes to get himself under control. By the time he returned, Lily had the table set and was pouring the wine.

"This looks amazing," he said.

They kept the conversation light over a salad garnished with olives and feta cheese, followed by lamb souvlaki with tzatziki.

"How long have you lived here?" Wolf asked.

"Almost seven years. Why?"

He glanced past the breakfast bar that separated the kitchen from the living room, taking in the sparsely furnished space. A couple armchairs, a coffee table, a modest wall-mounted flat-screen TV. Shelves crammed with textbooks and rows of loose leaf binders, their spines carefully labeled in block print. No photos or paintings on the walls, no plants in the corner, no throws draped over the sofa. All very neat. Impersonal.

"Just wondering," he said. "My place is a lot…messier."

She shrugged. "The cleaning service has my key. Even if I'm out or traveling, they make sure everything is taken care of. I deal with enough chaos out there—" she waved vaguely toward the door. "It would drive me nuts to have to deal with it when I come home."

He nodded and mopped up some tzatziki with a piece of pita. "You know what CDO is?"

"No, what?"

"OCD, with the letters alphabetized."

She blinked. "Are you calling me obsessive-compulsive?"

"Your binders are organized by size and color."

She followed his gaze to the bookcases lining the far wall. "No," she said. "They're actually organized according to project. White for studies. Black for conferences and workshops. Thinner binders for my notes. Thicker ones for supporting material or handouts."

"Of course." He wiped his fingers on a napkin. "How did I not know that?"

"You're making fun of me."

"Not at all. Some of my best friends are OCD. Take Doug's wife. She alphabetizes the spices. And counts everything. And I mean *everything*. Silverware, plates, glasses, napkins. Like she's still in the O.R., doing a sponge and needle count, where it actually matters if you're missing a sponge or two."

"She's a surgeon?"

"Scrub nurse. Or at least she used to be. Before she went back to school, got a master's in health administration, and worked her way up to Chief Nursing Officer at St. Mary's. You'd think at this point, she could delegate the counting, but no—" he raised a hand before Lily could object. "I know it doesn't work that way. Seriously. But I'm telling you, that woman is in for a shock once she wakes up and smells the dirty diapers. She's probably too wiped out to notice now, but in a few weeks' time, I bet you she'll realize that OCD and parenting just don't mix."

Lily pursed her lips. "That's ridiculous."

"Not at all. It's in the manual." He reached for the wine and topped up both their glasses. "Page two, paragraph three. In big bold letters: parenting and OCD don't mix."

"Right," she said. "Is that the OCD manual, or the parenting manual?"

"See, you're doing it again. Trying to nail it down." He shook his head. "Classic OCD."

"And you're trying to avoid answering the question. Classic PIA."

He laughed. How could he have thought this woman devoid of humor? "Just for the record, being a pain in the ass takes effort."

"And practice," she added. "I'm sure it takes lots and lots

of practice."

"Well, you keep talking about cultivating hobbies," he said. "Speaking of, what do you do for fun?"

She took a sip of wine. "I run. It doesn't require any special equipment. When you're on the road a lot, that's a huge plus."

"Do you do marathons, like your friend Parker?"

She studied him, as if puzzled by the sudden tightness in his voice. "No. I'm more of a 10K person. I've done a couple half-marathons, but it's tough to train for that when you travel so much. What about you? You play sports?"

He shrugged. "You name it, I've probably played it. But don't change the subject."

"What subject?"

"You and Parker."

"Really?" She raised a brow. "That's a subject?"

"You tell me. Are you seeing him?"

"Of course I see him. We're friends. We work on cases together."

Wolf dismissed her non-answer with a flick of the hand. "That's not what I'm asking. What I want to know is, are you sleeping with him?"

"Sleeping...with *Parker?*" Her mouth fell open. "Are you kidding me?"

He stiffened. "It's a serious question."

An immediate denial would have calmed his unexpected surge of jealousy.

Wolf wasn't the possessive type. He hated it when a woman got clingy. That was a sure sign the relationship was past its "sell by" date. And he was happy to offer his blessing to any woman he hooked up with who was ready to move on.

But the idea of Lily in some other guy's bed? *Hell, no.*

She smiled and shook her head. "I wouldn't be doing this—" she pointed at Wolf and then herself "—if I were sleeping with someone else."

"Okay. Good." Wolf forced his shoulders to relax. "I'm a free agent too."

"Glad we got that straightened out." She stood up and

started stacking empty plates. "Coffee?"

"Decaf if you have it." He helped her clear the table, then leaned back against the counter to watch her make the coffee. The hem of her shirt lifted as she reached overhead for the mugs, flashing a sliver of taut, smooth belly.

He gripped the edge of the counter behind him to keep from touching her. It would be all too easy to brush his fingers over that exposed skin, and follow the path of her ribs up beneath her shirt toward her breasts. He could almost feel the weight of them in his hands, nipples tightening as he stroked them through the bra.

But there was something he needed to clear up first, before he gave free rein to his fantasies.

"One more question," he said.

She glanced at him, eyes sweeping over the tense muscles of his shoulders and arms. He widened his stance, bringing her attention farther down, to the firm evidence of his arousal. Which only made him stiffen more.

She flushed and jerked her gaze back up. "Yes?"

"Who came up with the idea of calling Doug about the video?"

"Oh. He told you about that?"

"What did you expect?" He blew out a breath. "MD^2 is a joint venture. We don't do solo acts."

She bit her lip and turned back to the Keurig machine. The process of switching out mugs and replacing the used single-serve pod with a fresh one took an inordinate amount of attention. "I saw a few videos of you without Doug."

"He was probably behind the camera. In the early days, we couldn't afford to hire additional crew. We did everything ourselves."

"And now…?"

"The videos pay for themselves, thanks to ad revenue and a few strategic product placements."

"Advertisers must love you," she said. "All those millions of viewers."

He took a deep breath. "We do okay."

She slid one of the mugs his way. "Milk or sugar?"

"Just black."

She laced hers with milk. "Chocolate?"

"No, thanks." He watched as she opened the box, chose a truffle, and bit into it. Damn. As a stall tactic, this one bordered on cruel. His gaze zeroed in on the tiny smear of chocolate on her lower lip. She licked it off, and he nearly groaned.

No doubt about it. The woman was trying to kill him.

"So," she finally said. "What did you and Doug decide? About my—uh, Parker's idea?"

He clenched his jaw. "Still thinking about it."

"What will it take to convince you?"

Ah, there it was. Confirmation of that ugly little suspicion that had been plaguing him ever since she'd issued the dinner invitation.

Disappointment warred with anger.

And yet neither was a match for his driving desire to possess this woman.

Even if she'd lured him here under false pretenses and lulled him into believing that she was as hot for his body as he was for hers.

It didn't matter. He still wanted her. Wanted to explore every inch of her with his hands and mouth. Wanted her under him, over him, on the kitchen counter, up against the wall. Wanted her gasping his name as he pounded into her. Wanted to fuck her until neither of them could walk or talk or even think.

His hunger for her defied all logic. Sure, she was gorgeous and sexy. But there were plenty of other gorgeous, sexy women out there.

Women who didn't treat conversation as if it were a blood sport.

Women who would never presume to call him a Neanderthal.

Women who appreciated the difference between strength and weakness, and who didn't try to attack one while making excuses for the other.

"Wolf...?"

He shook his head to clear it. Then, just so there'd be no misunderstanding, he said it out loud. "Is that what tonight is all about? You wanted to seduce me into making your little video?"

Her eyes widened and she took a step back. "No."

"You sure?" he said, moving closer. "Because I'm not objecting to the seduction part. I'm just curious. How far were you willing to go to convince me?"

She frowned and took another step back. "You're twisting my words. I didn't mean..."

"What?" he said when she faltered. "You didn't mean what?"

"This has nothing to do with the video." Her gaze dropped to his lips, then slowly rose to meet his eyes. "I just...wanted to see you."

And just like that, his anger fizzled, leaving behind only raw, heart-pounding desire.

"In that case—" He closed the distance between them and cupped her jaw. Slowly, barely breathing, he kissed her.

She tasted of chocolate and coffee. Irresistible. He explored her mouth, while his fingers traced the contours of her cheek and jaw. Silky strands teased the back of his hand. He searched blindly for whatever was still keeping her hair confined and finally found the clip. Seconds later, it clattered to the floor. Her hair spilled over his hands and down her back, releasing the faint scent of berries. Plunging his fingers into the thick mass, he tugged lightly until she tilted her head back.

She gasped as his lips and tongue traced a slow path down her neck toward the madly pounding pulse at the base of her throat.

"Wolf..." Her fingers inched up around his shoulders, nails digging into the material when he nipped her skin. "Please..."

"Please, what...?"

Instead of answering, she pressed closer, arching her back, hips moving restlessly against him.

He abandoned her hair, and swept his hands down her spine, cupping her ass, lifting her.

She wrapped her legs around him. "My bedroom…"

"Where?"

She let go long enough to gesture toward the hall. And then her fingers were back, stroking up his arm, his shoulder, the back of his neck.

"Hang on."

She did, her breasts pressing against him, her legs tightening around his hips.

With each step his erection rubbed up against her. Even through multiple layers of clothing, he could feel her heat.

The faint spill of light from a street lamp just outside her bedroom window kept him from bumping into furniture. By the time they fell on the mattress, he was almost mindless with need. His mouth ravaged her lips, until they were both gasping for air.

But it wasn't enough.

Primed by two weeks of frustrated desire, he tugged at her clothing, his hands as clumsy and eager as a teenager's copping his first feel behind the school bleachers.

Lily helped, lifting her arms so he could peel off the lacy top, undoing the front closure of her bra. He pulled the cups apart, baring her breasts.

Perfect. Large enough to fill his hands, and exquisitely sensitive. The nipples pebbled beneath his touch as he kneaded and rolled them and then settled down to feast, licking and sucking until she was writhing beneath him.

He kissed his way down her stomach, pausing to unbutton, unzip, and then skim off her jeans, which left her in a whisper-thin thong.

"Wolf…" Her fingers tangled in his hair.

He breathed in her musky sweet scent. "You're wet for me, aren't you, baby?"

Her hips bucked, and she gasped as his fingers slipped beneath the silky fabric, parting her slick folds.

"Oh, yeah," he murmured. "Soaking wet."

A quick tug, and the thong was gone. He settled between her legs, lifting them up over his shoulders, leaving her wide open and completely at his mercy.

He traced the pad of his thumb around her clit, not quite touching, and when she moaned and raised her hips, he lowered his mouth and traced the same path with his tongue.

Her thighs quivered. Fingernails dug into his scalp. He ignored the pain and sank a finger into her tight heat, all the while licking and sucking on her clit. Another finger joined the first.

Her muscles clenched around him as he continued the dual assault with his hand and mouth, and before long she was crying out, hips jerking against him, internal muscles contracting around his fingers.

He almost lost it. The sight of her climaxing, and the knowledge that he'd been the one to bring her to this point, was nearly enough to make him come. But he wanted more. He wanted to bury himself deep inside her, again and again, until she was convulsing around him, driving them both over the edge.

He eased her down atop the duvet cover and slid off the bed. For a long moment he simply stood there, heart hammering, cock straining against the stiff material of his jeans, every muscle drawn and ready for action.

"Mm." Lily stirred and opened her eyes. When she caught sight of him, her lips curved up and she stretched. Slowly. Languorously. Arms raised above her head, back arched, her breasts on prominent display, she looked like some pagan sex goddess.

Wolf stared at her, hardly daring to breathe, let alone move, for fear that she would disappear like a lust-induced illusion.

Instead of disappearing, she sat up and swept her fingers through her hair.

Wolf watched, mesmerized, as she twisted the heavy mass into some semblance of order and draped it over one shoulder, where it partially covered her breast. The nipple poked through, a hard little nubbin that drew his attention and robbed him of the ability to string two words together.

Lily seemed to have no such difficulty. "You're still dressed," she said. Her gaze flickered down to the unmistakable bulge at his groin and then back up to his face. "Going somewhere?"

He cleared his throat and managed a single word. "No."

And then he started to strip. Fumbling for a condom from his wallet, he rolled it on, his cock swelling even more beneath her fascinated gaze.

She licked her lips and reached for him. "My turn."

The thought of that mouth on him, sucking him off, was almost too much to bear.

"Next time," he growled, removing her hand and kissing the palm. For now, he was too close to spontaneous combustion to take any more stimulation.

The mattress dipped beneath his weight. He followed Lily down, unceremoniously claiming her mouth and nudging her thighs apart. She was tight and wet and so ready that he slid into her with one smooth stroke, stopping only when he was seated to the hilt. She moved beneath him, urging him into an ever-accelerating rhythm punctuated by soft gasps and the slap of flesh against flesh.

He lost track of time. Everything became a blur. A frantic, glorious, dazzling rush of heat and movement and pleasure so intense that every nerve in his body tingled with the aftershocks.

Somehow—minutes? hours? later—he managed to drag himself away from Lily's seductive warmth with the mumbled excuse of needing to be in the hospital early the following morning.

He was dressed and halfway home when he realized he would much rather have stayed the night in Lily's bed.

The thought set off alarm bells.

He *never* stayed the night. It set up expectations he had no intention of pursuing.

He'd spent his entire childhood dreaming of escape. From the tiny bedroom he'd shared with his older brother, and the single bathroom where someone was always banging on the door, and the hot water inevitably ran out too soon. From the weight of responsibility they'd all had to assume even before hitting puberty, because their father was too ill, and then dead, and their mother couldn't manage four boys alone on a teacher's salary.

Too many people crammed into too little space left him feeling resentful and hemmed in.

Sure, he loved his family, and he did his share of mowing lawns and caddying and tutoring to keep the fridge stocked and SoCal Edison from shutting off the power.

But he still couldn't wait to break free.

It took years. Studying and working nights through college while his friends partied. Powering through biochemistry and gross anatomy, while med school classmates complained about exams being too tough, and why weren't they graded on a curve? Moonlighting in an inner city ER where every third patient arrived with a gunshot or stab wound, while fellow residents groaned about the demands of treating the worried well.

He could have given up at any point. Decided it was too much, too hard, not worth the trouble. But he persevered. Because he was never going back to the hand-to-mouth existence of his childhood.

And in the end, he'd succeeded. Not through any handouts or entitlements or loopholes in the system, but through years of hard work and determination and refusing to give up.

Now he had his own place. Enough money to pay off his student loans and mortgage—and set his mother up in a comfortable house with the nine-foot Steinway grand she'd always wanted but could never afford.

He had a career he loved, and a side gig that was both entertaining and financially rewarding. There was time to surf and hike and play hockey every other Sunday. And he never lacked for female company.

Things were just how he wanted, and he planned on keeping it that way.

No way was he going to let anything—or anyone—jeopardize the lifestyle he'd worked so hard to achieve.

Which was why the idea of spending an entire night with a woman, of *sleeping* with her as opposed to just having sex and leaving, scared the shit out of him. He didn't need that kind of trouble. Didn't want the responsibility of caring for someone else.

And if he ever doubted the slippery slope argument, all he had to do was look at Doug. The poor bastard had gone from playboy to parent in less than a year. That's what happened when you let down your guard.

But even that reminder wasn't enough to keep him from dreaming about Lily.

Not that night. Or the night after. Or the night after that.

CHAPTER SIX

"When are you back in town?" Wolf asked a week later, when they'd finally managed to connect by phone.

Texts and emails were safe, undemanding.

They fit into his schedule, now that he was back in the hospital for seven days straight, working twelve to fourteen hour shifts.

And they accommodated Lily's travel schedule. She left mid-week for a four-day conference in D.C.

But Wolf missed her, dammit.

Emojis were no substitute for hearing the laughter in her voice or sinking into the welcoming warmth of her embrace.

"Next Saturday," she said.

Next Saturday? As in, another eight days away? "I thought your conference ends tomorrow."

"It does," she said. "But since I'm already in D.C., I set up some meetings with colleagues here in town."

Fuck. He'd been looking forward to seeing her during his week off. For days he'd been distracted with thoughts of her. While standing in line at the hospital cafeteria. Or in the rare quiet moment seated in the physician lounge. Or when tossing in bed, recalling the way she tasted, and how her entire body tensed and then went limp the first time he'd made her come.

Now it looked like she wasn't planning to return until he was back on service.

Maybe he could trade a few days with one of the other hospitalists. Free up the weekend Lily was back so he could take her to bed and keep her there until they were both too tired to move. He needed some kind of recompense for this prolonged and decidedly uncomfortable stretch of abstinence.

He was in the emergency room, doing an admission later that day, when an altercation erupted outside one of the exam cubicles.

"Out of my way, bitch—"

"Sir, you need to calm down," a female voice responded. Rachel Harding, one of the ER docs.

Fuck.

Rachel was pregnant and looked like she was about to pop any second. Wolf didn't know her well, but her husband was the head of surgery. He'd been one of Wolf's mentors when Wolf first joined St. Mary's fresh out of residency.

Wolf headed toward the raised voices, pulling the stethoscope from his neck and tossing it aside as he went.

"Call security," he barked as he strode past the nurses' station.

"You telling me what to do, bitch?" The man towered over Rachel, hands twitching. Even from fifteen feet away, Wolf could smell him: the stale stench of sweat and cat urine. "I'll cut you like I cut that fucking whore—"

Around them, all activity had stopped. Nurses, orderlies, clerks, and even patients lying on gurneys along the wall, remained frozen in place as they watched the scene unfold.

"Please, sir," Rachel said, slowly edging back. Her hands hovered protectively over her stomach. "I'm sure we can work this out."

Wolf grabbed the closest thing to a weapon he could find— a dirty linen cart—and shoved it into the man's side. The impact sent the guy sprawling, but not for long.

Wolf shrugged off his white coat and tossed it aside. From the corner of his eye, he saw Rachel slipping past him, out of harm's way. *Good girl.*

The man was already scrambling to his feet, cursing and fumbling in the pocket of his jacket.

Wolf didn't hesitate. He pushed aside the cart, grabbed the man by the front flaps of his jacket, and took him down with a single-leg sweep.

The move spurred others into action. A couple orderlies rushed forward to help. Between the three of them, they managed to secure the man, who continued to thrash on the ground and spew obscenities.

Security arrived and took over. Within minutes, the police were there as well.

Wolf exchanged a few words with one of the officers, then left them to it.

As he disinfected his hands with gel from one of the ubiquitous wall dispensers, staff members filed by to offer quick pats on the back.

A medical assistant returned his white coat. One of the LVN's retrieved his stethoscope.

Slowly, everyone drifted back to work.

Wolf found Rachel slumped in a chair behind the nurses' station. Her face was still as white as her coat. Someone had gotten her a cup of tea, but it stood untouched in front of her.

"You okay?" He snagged a nearby chair and sat down beside her.

She blinked and glanced up. "Thanks for the rescue."

"All in a day's work."

She offered a shaky laugh. "They don't teach moves like that in med school."

"They do in Krav Maga." At her blank look, he said, "Israeli defense fighting."

"Ah." She nodded and fell silent.

Wolf's phone pinged. He glanced at the message: one of the hospital case managers letting him know that there were still no skilled nursing facility beds available for a patient he'd been trying to transfer since yesterday.

Great, just what he needed.

The next call would no doubt be from some utilization review person, asking why the patient was still in the hospital.

Fucking bureaucrats.

"If you have to get that, go ahead." Rachel said, nodding toward his cell. "You don't need to hold my hand."

He shrugged. "It can wait. You want me to call someone for you? Your husband?"

"No." She glanced at the clock. "He's probably still in surgery. I'm sure he'll hear all about it once he finishes the case. You know the crazy thing about this?"

"What?"

"We argued just yesterday. Erik doesn't want me working."

"Well, the ER isn't exactly the safest place." Wolf's eyes dropped to her massive belly. "You know, considering."

"Yeah," she sighed. "The guy attacked his girlfriend with a knife. Lucky for her, his aim was off. She got away and had a neighbor bring her in."

"Was she badly hurt?"

"A few lacerations. The longest was twelve centimeters. No blood vessel or tendon involvement, so we boostered her tetanus, gave her a shot of Rocephin, and did a double layer closure. I'd just paged social work when the boyfriend showed up."

"You think she'll press charges?"

Rachel shook her head. "Doubt it. She's one of our regulars. Goes back to him every time. Because he *loves* her. He loves her so much that one of these days he's going to kill her."

Wolf frowned. He was familiar with the grim statistics on domestic violence. His brother Joe's wife worked as a therapist and volunteered at a local shelter. Every year, she helped organize a big fundraiser for the cause, and hit Wolf up for a hefty donation.

"Maybe if she knew she had options—"

"I've talked with her before," Rachel said. "So have the social workers. I don't know, maybe this time they'll manage to get through to her..."

Wolf narrowed his eyes. "What about you? He assaulted you—"

"He *threatened* me."

"Close enough. Isn't that worth some jail time?"

"Oh, sure. *If* he's convicted. He'll be out in six months, maybe a year if they manage to get him on drug possession. It's obvious he's using, but unless he has some crystal meth or drug paraphernalia on him…" She shrugged. "The county jails are overcrowded. There are bigger fish to fry. Trust me, I've been through this before."

Wolf hesitated. "Maybe you should listen to Erik and go on maternity leave."

"Maybe. Though I'm not due for another three months. I know," she smiled and rubbed her belly. "Hard to believe, right? We had trouble getting pregnant. I'm forty. Erik's…well, older. He already has kids from his first marriage. They're in college now. He wasn't too keen about starting over, but I managed to convince him. The nice thing about living on the Westside is there's no shortage of fertility clinics. So, twins."

"Oh. Well, congratulations."

"Thanks." She looked up as one of the police officers approached.

Wolf rose. "I should get going, finish admitting my patient. You'll be okay?"

"Like you said, all in a day's work."

Several hours later, Wolf leaned against the wall in one of the stairwells and closed his eyes.

He'd just spent forty-five minutes explaining to the family of a patient dying from metastatic lung cancer why aggressive intervention at this point was medically futile. The man had bone, liver, and brain mets, and had failed multiple rounds of chemo, radiation, and immunotherapy. Comfort care was the only reasonable and humane option.

But one of the children insisted on another oncology and pulmonary consult, and there was nothing Wolf could do but go along with the request, and order a medical ethics consult along with it.

If he had to fight the family on this, he would, though he hated doing it.

The process of going through official channels, requesting a formal hearing in front of the hospital's medical ethics committee, presenting his case, and waiting for the committee's written determination, only prolonged his patient's suffering.

But unless the family agreed to palliative care or hospice, Wolf's hands were tied. He had to do everything by the book or risk getting sued.

Why couldn't people accept that some conditions were simply not curable, or even treatable?

People got sick. People died. That was reality.

Wolf rubbed his eyes and took a deep breath.

Despite changing into fresh scrubs after his confrontation with the meth head, and using a boatload of disinfectant gel since then, he still felt grimy.

What he needed was a long hot shower and a few solid days of sleep.

And sex. The kind that blew your mind and wrung you out and had you coming back for more.

Except Lily was out of town, and wouldn't be back for another week.

And he still had evening rounds and sign-out to get through.

For once, he wasn't sure he'd make it. Exhaustion weighed down his limbs and seeped through his pores like some invisible toxin.

In his mind's eye, he could see Doug's conveyor belt. Could feel it moving beneath his feet.

And there, in the distance, just as Doug described, loomed the massive meat grinder.

Wolf swayed, felt himself falling.

Down, down, down he went, until he was back in the ER, walking along an endless hallway lined with gurneys. There were patients lying on those gurneys, and they moaned as he passed by, their ghostly arms reaching out, skeletal fingers clutching at his sleeves. One by one, they rose to follow him. Like a white-coated Pied Piper, Wolf led his entourage toward a door at the end of the hall.

The door opened into a call room. Desk, chair, lockers. Bunk beds, filled with interns in scrubs. The phone rang, and each intern popped up, like a jack-in-the-box.

But the phone kept ringing, and Wolf jerked awake to discover his own phone buzzing and vibrating at his waist. He stared at the gray cement walls of the hospital stairwell, appalled that for the first time in his life he'd fallen asleep on the job.

It was a miracle that he'd remained on his feet, propped against the wall.

He scrubbed a hand down his face, the two-day-old bristles scratching his palm.

Then he straightened up and answered the phone.

Because he was strong, dammit. And he didn't believe in burnout.

CHAPTER SEVEN

By Monday evening, Lily realized she'd made a mistake in staying an extra week.

D.C. in October was dark, wet, and dreary.

Her body was still on West Coast time, so dragging herself out of bed to go running at dawn didn't appeal. And by the time her meetings were over, it was dark. Which meant her only option was the treadmill at the hotel gym.

She was just hitting her stride when her phone rang.

She glanced at the display. Wolf.

Smiling, she switched off the music and hit the button to decrease her speed. "Hi."

A moment of silence greeted her. And then Wolf's voice, uncharacteristically cautious, "Am I interrupting something?"

"My eight-minute mile," she said. "But that's okay. I can slow down. Jog and talk at the same time."

"Oh. Where are you?"

"Hotel gym." She slowed her pace even more. "I'm not big on gyms. But this one's not bad. The treadmills are in good shape. Nice shock absorption. I haven't tried the salt water pool yet. Or the sauna. Maybe tomorrow."

He groaned. "You're doing this on purpose, aren't you?"

"What?"

"Getting me all hot and bothered. When I can't do anything about it."

She flushed at the image those words evoked. "I'm sure you can do *something* about it."

"Mm. Yeah. Maybe." A long pause. "But doing it alone…isn't as much…fun."

Now *he* sounded out of breath.

Was he…? Oh, my.

She stumbled and nearly went down as she pictured him lying in bed. Naked.

Oh yes, definitely naked. And fully aroused. One hand holding the phone, the other wrapped around his very…impressive…erection. Stroking. Slowly. From the thick base all the way to the engorged head, and then back down again.

She hit the emergency stop button and grabbed the handlebars to keep herself from falling. "Wolf?"

"Mm-hm."

"What are you doing?"

"Imagining you here. With me."

She licked her lips and glanced around.

There were a half dozen other guests using various pieces of equipment. Thankfully, none of them seemed to be paying her any attention.

Even so, she lowered her voice. "Listen, can I call you back? I need to…uh…go. To my room. To cool off."

His husky laughter swept across her skin like a hot breath. "You do that, baby."

Sweat trickled down the back of her neck and dampened the fabric between her breasts. So much for "moisture-wicking technology."

She gathered her water bottle, phone, and keycard, and dropped off her used towel in the bin by the door.

It took fifteen minutes to shower, dry her hair, and slip on some boxers and an ancient UCSD T-shirt.

She climbed into bed and picked up the phone.

Wolf answered on the first ring. "Feeling better?"

"Yes," she said. "You?"

"I'm okay. How's D.C.?"

"Lonely." *Oops.* That wasn't what she'd meant to say. She closed her eyes and tried again. "I'm getting a lot done. Today I met this professor from Georgetown who's looking at the effect of reduced resident work hours on clinical outcomes..."

She launched into a detailed explanation of the professor's findings, hoping to bury her gaffe beneath an avalanche of words.

It didn't work.

"Lily."

"Yes?"

"I'm free for the rest of the week," he said. "And I haven't been to D.C. in years. What do you say I fly out for a couple days? I'll play tourist while you work. Then at night we can go out. Or stay in. Your call."

If he'd said that Martians were landing outside her hotel, she might have recovered more quickly, and offered a more intelligent comeback than: "Why?"

"Because I've had a rough week," he said, apparently unfazed by her unenthusiastic response. "I could use some time away, and there's lots to do in D.C. Walk around the National Mall—"

"It's raining," she blurted. "This whole week."

"Okay, so something indoors. One of the Smithsonian museums. I wonder if they still have the interactive flight simulator at the Air & Space museum?"

"I don't know. I've never been."

"You're kidding," he said. "Never?"

"When I come to D.C., it's for work."

"Oh, baby, you are so missing out. But don't worry, we'll fix that. How about you take a day off and go with me?"

"I can't."

"Why not?"

Lily took a deep breath. "Because people went out of their way to rearrange their schedules so they could meet with me. I'm not going to abuse their goodwill and renege on my commitments in order to play hooky with you."

"Ouch. Well, at least now I know where I stand in the pecking order."

She bit her lip. "Are you mad?"

"No, I'm not mad." He paused. "But maybe I'm being presumptuous. Do you even want me there?"

"I can't believe we're discussing this," she said. "It's crazy. I mean, I'll be back Saturday. We can see each other then. Why fly three thousand miles for a couple days when you don't have to?"

"Hm, when you put it that way, I guess you're right. It does sound crazy."

She should have kept her mouth shut. *Stupid, stupid, stupid.* So what if the idea of Wolf joining her in D.C. wasn't practical or even sane?

He was the first man to capture her attention and spark her libido in longer than she cared to remember. The first man ever to give her multiple orgasms.

And he was offering to hop a plane and travel cross-country on the spur of the moment just to be with her.

What was she thinking, turning him down?

"Wolf—"

"Lily—"

She swallowed a bubble of nervous laughter. "I'm staying at the Fairmont in Georgetown."

"The Fairmont," he repeated. "Georgetown. Okay, got it. Do I need to book a separate room?"

"No." She closed her eyes and let out the breath she hadn't even realized she was holding.

"Great. I'll text you the details once I've booked a flight. And Lily?"

"Yes?"

"Get some sleep while you can."

Oh, My God.

He booked a red-eye for Wednesday evening, arriving in Dulles airport at seven-thirty the following morning.

After texting Lily the details, he started having second thoughts.

Two days and nights, sharing a hotel room. Christ, she'd have them engaged and married by the end of the weekend. What the fuck had he been thinking?

That was the problem. He hadn't been thinking. At least not with his brain.

All it took was hearing her breathy voice, and his imagination was off and running. Lily, in skimpy workout gear. Or a teeny bikini. Or completely naked, spread out on a bed, waiting. For him.

Because she was *lonely*.

It was that soft confession that did it, not to mention her cheeky suggestion that he jerk off to relieve his sexual frustration.

He had.

But the moment she was back on the phone he was hard as ever, cursing the distance between them.

So, yeah, he wanted to see her. But maybe she was right. Maybe waiting until she returned to L.A. was a better move.

He pulled up the airline website on his phone. Re-read the fine print on his ticket. Non-transferable, non-refundable.

Fuck.

So either he threw away the money already spent, and went through another five miserable days of waiting, or he ponied up a few hundred more per night and got a separate hotel room. A place where he could dump his stuff and retreat after sating his appetite with Lily.

He chose option number two. If she asked, he could always come up with an excuse. He didn't want to crowd her. Or he was a night owl, and had work to do on the computer. Whatever.

Arrangements made, Wolf threw together a travel bag, then did the one thing guaranteed to drown out whatever doubts remained: he headed for his studio.

It had taken the better part of a year to convert the garage into a soundproofed space equipped with everything he and Doug needed to record, edit, and mix their soundtracks.

When he couldn't sleep, the studio was his refuge.

After a few hours of experimenting, he called Doug. "I need your help."

Doug yawned. "With what?"

"Did I wake you?" Wolf glanced at the time display at the corner of his computer screen. Past midnight. "Sorry. Never mind, this can wait till morning."

Another yawn. Then, "I'm back to work this week. So now's better than morning. What's up?"

"I need the lyrics."

"What lyrics?"

"The ones you were working on." Wolf made another notation on the sheet music he'd downloaded earlier. "You know, *We don't need your innovation...*"

"But you said—"

"I know what I said. Just send me the lyrics, okay?"

"What changed your mind?"

"Nothing changed my mind." He tapped the pencil against his jean-clad thigh. "I'm still thinking."

"But you want the lyrics."

"Yes."

"They're not done."

"Send me whatever you have."

"Okay. Give me a few minutes."

"Thanks." Wolf put his headphones back on and switched from recording the piano part to the virtual guitar.

He'd put the tracks together later. Piano, guitar, bass, drums. Once that was edited, he and Doug could work on the vocals.

The storyboard usually came later, after the soundtrack was done. He'd listen to the music on endless repeat while planning out the scenes.

This time, though, everything seemed to be jumbled in his head. Images flashed across his brain, entire sequences that made his fingers itch to pick up a pencil and start sketching.

He'd work on it tomorrow. And maybe in D.C., while Lily was off taking meetings.

Not that he was committing to anything. A storyboard and soundtrack were just the beginning. He could decide at any point to pull the plug.

And even if they did make the video, there was no guarantee Lily would like it.

But at the moment, none of that mattered. There was only the music, wrapping itself around him like a dream.

CHAPTER EIGHT

Lily couldn't believe he was here.

Sure, he'd texted her the flight information. But even then she thought he'd change his mind, or something would come up, and she'd be left more frustrated than she had been before he brought up the possibility of joining her in D.C.

But Wolf did more than just keep his promise to show up.

He appointed himself entertainment director, whisking her off on a private moonlit tour of the capital with a hired driver/guide. Dinner followed at an intimate jazz club, where the singer performed such an uncanny rendition of Ella Fitzgerald's "How High the Moon" that Lily could swear she was listening to the Queen of Jazz herself.

Back at the hotel, Lily sighed and rested her head on Wolf's bare shoulder. The scent of night rain and sex hung in the air.

"We should close the windows," she murmured, idly tracing the whorls of hair on his chest to where they bisected his abs.

He caught her fingers before they wandered farther south. "Later."

She fell asleep before *later* came, and woke up to an empty bed and watery sunlight filtering around the edges of the black-out curtains.

For a moment she wondered where Wolf was. And then she remembered.

He'd reserved his own room.

"I'm a restless sleeper," he'd said, when she questioned his lack of luggage. "I figured the least I could do was get out of your way so you could get some sleep. Since you're working and all."

How kind and thoughtful of him.

And how utterly full of shit.

She knew a fellow commitment-phobe when she saw one.

The signs were unmistakable. Like the eye-roll that accompanied his description of Doug's newfound domesticity. And his choice of car. A red two-seater. Could it get any more clichéd than that?

And yet Wolf was the one who'd engineered this rendezvous, traveling long-distance and at considerable expense to spend time with her.

Which meant…what?

She thought about it as she showered and prepared for another day of meetings.

Not that it mattered. She wasn't on the market for anything more than some good—make that great—sex and fun times, which Wolf was both willing and able to provide. His methods might be a little over-the-top, but he still seemed as leery of entanglement as she was.

So, no need to stress. She should just relax and enjoy whatever he had planned for the evening.

It turned out to be a dinner cruise along the Potomac River. After the meal, they danced to the mellow strains of Cole Porter and the soft pitter-patter of rain on the glass-enclosed deck.

During a set break, they returned to their table for coffee and a shared plate of miniature pastries.

Lily licked the cream off her spoon. "This raspberry mousse is amazing. You should try it."

He leaned in and brushed his thumb over her lower lip, where a trace of mousse remained.

"Mm," he said, licking the remnants off his finger. "You're right. I think I need another taste."

Her eyes widened, but before she could get a word out, his mouth covered hers.

Oh, this was *way* better than raspberry mousse.

The spoon dropped from her nerveless fingers. Her lids drifted shut. She was floating, weightless, tethered only by Wolf's lips and hands, which seemed to be everywhere at once, stroking her cheek and jaw, angling her head for better access, tracing the delicate skin of her neck.

In the background, the low hum of conversation and soft clink of silverware against glass faded to nothing.

Breathing became optional.

It was Wolf who finally pulled away. "Lily."

She smiled dreamily, swaying to the music in her head.

"The band is back," Wolf said.

Her eyes fluttered open. Sure enough, the dance floor was starting to fill up again.

She glanced at Wolf. "You want to…?"

"In a minute." He shifted in his seat. "I miscalculated."

"How so?"

"We're stuck, at least for a while. And there are no rooms for rent." His lips quirked. "Unless you want to make a quick trip to the restroom to…check out the facilities?"

Her nose wrinkled. Sex in a public bathroom? The ick factor alone was enough to put her off the idea. "Have you ever…?"

"Sure," he said. "In residency, you don't have time to be too fussy. You take what you can get whenever and wherever you can get it."

"Sounds like a breeding ground for STD's."

He shrugged. "Nothing a shot of Rocephin can't cure."

Her mouth fell open.

"Kidding," he laughed. "Sorry, your expression…I couldn't resist. Anyway, you have nothing to worry about. I'm always careful. Especially in public restrooms. Doctors' creed, right?"

"Maybe we should use a double-layer of protection. You

know, just in case."

"Oh, come on, Lil, I was joking."

"Which part was the joke?"

He reached for her hand. "You're not upset, are you?"

She shrugged. "Around you, I'm never sure what to think."

"At least you're not bored."

"No," she said. "I'm not bored."

Wolf snagged a seat next to Lily on the flight back, thanks to another passenger who was willing to trade.

"I can't believe she fell for it," Lily murmured after takeoff. "*Young couple in love*, my ass."

"Ooh, I love it when you talk dirty," he laughed.

She shook her head and pulled out her computer. "I've got some work to do."

"All work and no play—"

"We had plenty of play time the last few days," she said.

"But we could always use more." He leaned in, lips against her ear. "Wanna try for the mile-high club?"

She flushed, glad they were in a two-seat row. Hopefully no one in the rows in front or behind them had supersonic hearing.

Just in case, she lowered her voice. "I thought we'd settled that whole sex-in-public-places thing."

"I didn't realize you meant it as a blanket statement." He grunted obligingly as she elbowed him in the ribs. "Okay, okay, I hear you. But you can't blame a guy for trying."

He waited until the flight attendants wheeling the beverage cart moved down the aisle, then extracted his own computer from an overhead compartment.

Over the next hour, Lily's eyes kept straying from her computer screen to Wolf's. Finally, curiosity got the better of her. "What are you doing?"

He glanced up from the tablet. "Storyboard. For a new video."

"Oh." She squinted at what looked like a handout page from one of her PowerPoint presentations. Or would have looked like it, if her slides had stick figure drawings with arrows pointing every which way and comments scrawled in indecipherable code on the side. "What's the video about?"

"It's a secret." He drew his thumb and index finger across the seam of his lips, miming a zipper closing. "At least until I figure out if we'll actually do it."

"And the storyboard helps you decide?"

"Sometimes. At the very least, it helps to visualize the story. When you map out the scenes, it's easier to see what works, what doesn't." He scrolled forward a few pages, then zoomed in on a single box. "Here, you see? Each frame shows a new action or shot. These arrows tell you which way the character's moving. And the arrows here along the outside describe the camera movement."

She tilted her head, but the markings still looked like chicken scratch to her.

"Think of it as a comic strip," Wolf said. When she didn't respond, he glanced at her. "You know, like the comics in the Sunday paper. Peanuts, Garfield, Doonesbury…"

"Sorry," she shrugged. "Not my usual reading material."

"But surely as kid…?"

"No." She could just picture her father's response. *Reids do not read garbage.* "My dad was…how should I put it? Strict."

Wolf frowned. "What do you mean?"

"He's a perfectionist. Everything has to be just right, according to his standards." She saved the file she was working on and shut down her computer. "And if, God forbid, you fail to measure up…well, let's just say, things could get very unpleasant."

Wolf's hand settled over hers. "Unpleasant, how?"

"Oh, he's not violent," Lily said quickly. "But the way he rips into you when you've done something wrong—or something he perceives as wrong—makes you feel about an inch tall. When he's *really* mad, he doesn't say anything at all. Just ignores you, like you're not even there. I spent a lot of my childhood either being invisible, or wishing I were."

Wolf brushed his thumb across her knuckles. "He sounds like a miserable human being."

"Not always. He's very charismatic when he wants to be. Patients love him."

"He's a doctor?"

"Cardiothoracic surgeon."

Wolf's thumb stilled. "Wait a minute. *Reid.* Frederick Reid? That's your father?"

"Yes. You know him?"

"Not personally. But I know *of* him. I have patients with ICDs that he patented. He pretty much cornered the market on implantable cardioverter defibrillators."

"If you don't count Medtronic and Boston Scientific, then yes."

"Shit. Why didn't you say something?" He released her hand and busied himself with shutting down and putting away his tablet.

She watched in silence as he pulled out a set of noise-canceling headphones and settled back in his seat. It wasn't until he started to put on the headphones that she reached out and stayed his hand. "I didn't realize it was such a big deal."

"Are you kidding me?" He looked at her, brows drawn. "You let me go on and on about what it takes to be a doctor. Without ever once mentioning that you grew up with *Frederick* fucking *Reid.*"

"I still don't see the problem."

His eyes narrowed. "It's like me telling Bill Gates' kid what it's like to build a computer. You must have been laughing the whole time."

"I wasn't laughing. And what I know about being a doctor has nothing to do with my father."

"Right. Because you stuck it out and went into medicine yourself."

She let go of his hand and gripped the armrest. Hard. "Wolf—"

"No wonder you felt free to drop out when things got

tough. Unlike those of us who actually have to work for a living, you've got Daddy's billions to fall back on. You can afford to look for some kind of abstract *meaning* in medicine."

She closed her eyes and blew out a breath. Since that first dinner at her place, when Wolf left in a huff, they'd avoided discussing the specifics of her work. Sex was obviously a powerful motivator. But it wasn't enough to plaster over their fundamental differences. Whatever temporary truce they'd achieved already seemed to be breaking down.

She opened her eyes and saw that he'd put the headphones on. Ha. Like that was going to stop her. She grabbed the earpiece closest to her and lifted. "So you're mad at me because of my dad's money?"

He slid the headphones off, leaving them around his neck. A muscle ticked in his jaw. "No. Not exactly."

"Then what?"

"You want to know what pisses me off?" He gripped their shared armrest and leaned closer. "It's when people with no understanding of reality presume to lecture the rest of us on how things ought to be."

"And by 'people' you mean me?"

"If the shoe fits, princess."

"Well, it doesn't," she said. "I can tell you all about reality. It's a twenty-seven year old OB/gyn resident with Hodgkin's lymphoma who's refused time off for chemo and radiation. When she protests, she's called a slacker and troublemaker, gets scathing evaluations, and is ultimately fired. This is someone who's always been top of her class and consistently received glowing reviews from her attendings—including those who later dumped on her when she got sick. *That's* reality."

"If that actually happened—"

"There's no *if* about it," she said. "The woman wrote to me because she'd heard me speak. When she told me her story, I set her up with a lawyer, and the case is going through the courts right now."

"There are two sides to every story." Wolf held up his hand to keep her from interrupting again. "Like I said, *if* it happened the way this woman said it did, then that's terrible. But you don't condemn an entire system because of one or two outliers."

"That's the problem," she said. "This isn't an outlier. For every physician whose case I've personally gotten involved in, there are hundreds more just like it."

He sighed. "Lily—"

"No," she said. "*This* is reality. Brushing it off or ignoring it won't make it go away. And if you think this kind of abuse doesn't happen every day, then *you're* the one who has no understanding of reality."

"Look, I don't want to argue—"

"Fine," she said. "Then don't."

They lapsed into silence.

The meal service came and went.

Lily excused herself to use the restroom. As she washed her hands, she glanced around the tiny cubicle and tried to work out the logistics of sex at thirty-six thousand feet.

Though considering where she and Wolf had left things, she doubted there'd be any sex at all, regardless of location.

When they landed and Wolf offered to share a taxi, she felt a brief flare of hope. Maybe she'd misread the situation.

"Look," Wolf said, as they sat in traffic. "We had a good time, right?"

"Yes."

"And even if we disagree, we can still be friends."

Lily swallowed and forced a smile. "Sure. Friends."

There were worse things than being friendzoned.

All she had to do was turn on the news. War. Famine. Destruction wrought by all kinds of natural and man-made disasters.

"Can you wait a minute?" Wolf said to the driver.

She blinked. When had they gotten home?

"As long as the meter's running," the driver said. "I can wait all day. You need help with the luggage?"

Lily opened the door. "Yes—"

"No—" Wolf exited the other side.

They met at the open trunk.

"I've got it," Lily said.

But Wolf was already lifting her suitcase and computer bag out, wheeling them toward the entrance to her building.

She hurried after him. "I can take it from here."

"You sure?"

"Yes. Thanks."

He nodded and started to walk away, then turned back. "Lily."

"Yes—"

Whatever she'd been about to say got lost when his mouth covered hers.

Oh, yes.

His arm around her waist was the only thing keeping her upright.

And then, as abruptly as it started, the kiss ended.

"I'll call you," he said.

She sank down atop her suitcase—thankfully a rugged model with a hard polycarbonate shell—and watched the taxi pull away.

CHAPTER NINE

Plan A—getting together with Lily for Sunday brunch—fell through.

Who knew that a healthcare policy consultant/motivational speaker—or whatever she chose to call herself—could get tagged for an emergency consult?

"I'm sorry," Lily told him over the phone. "Something's come up and I have to go downtown. Can we reschedule for another day?"

"I'm on service this week," Wolf said. "It'll be crazy."

"Next weekend then." A door slammed. "We'll figure it out."

"There's no way you can postpone this downtown thing till Monday?" Wolf said.

"No." Her voice sounded clipped and considerably cooler than it had just minutes ago. "It can't wait till Monday."

Which was how Wolf ended up spending the rest of his weekend at Doug and Tina's.

In between diaper changes and trading off baby care with his wife, Doug helped finalize the lyrics and hash out the storyline.

"When are you free to record?" Wolf said, packing up his computer and portable midi keyboard.

Doug flopped back on the couch and yawned. "I don't know."

"How about next weekend?" A few hours to record the vocals, and he'd still have the rest of the day to do...whatever. The mixing and mastering he could do on his own, anytime.

Doug blinked. "You have two weekends off in a row?"

"Yeah," Wolf said. "It happens. So do I book the sound guy?"

"Let me check with Tina. I'll get back to you."

On the way home, Wolf stopped by his favorite Chinese restaurant. As he waited for the takeout order, he pulled out his phone and checked for messages. Nothing in the last few hours, since Lily's last reply: *Still working. Talk later.*

He resisted the urge to text her. Was she really working, or simply brushing him off?

Before meeting Lily, he'd never obsessed over a woman's motivations. Women simply didn't keep him hanging. And if they tried to play mind games, he cut them loose without a qualm. Life was too short for that kind of shit.

But there was something about Lily that kept drawing him back. Something beyond the physical attraction and the visceral, atavistic response of his body to hers. Was it her intelligence and dry sense of humor? Or her altruism and dedication to righting perceived wrongs?

He didn't agree with her views, but he had to admire her discipline and courage in tackling issues that few others would touch. She was either delusional in thinking she could take on the establishment, or simply didn't care that by attacking the foundations on which physician training and practice were based, she'd make herself a pariah in the medical community.

Was that why she left residency? Had she already made enemies within her program, and been forced out as a result?

Or had she embarked on a campaign to reform the system only after dropping out?

In either case, Wolf conceded that her failure to complete residency had nothing to do with intelligence. That, she had in spades.

And she wasn't a slacker, despite his initial assumptions. In fact, she worked harder than some of the doctors he knew.

Wolf's phone pinged with an incoming text from Doug: *Green light for Saturday.*

Excellent. A brief exchange with the sound engineer whom they typically used, and they were set.

At home, Wolf kicked off his shoes, dumped his computer bag and keyboard, and ate beef and broccoli straight from the container while watching the evening news.

The usual lineup of political idiocy, human misery, and frivolous celebrity gossip.

He was about to switch channels when a breaking news alert caught his attention. He turned up the volume.

"—update on a story we've been following about a body found earlier today in Boyle Heights, in an apartment building just half a mile from the USC Health Sciences campus.

"The man, who died in an apparent suicide, has been identified as Brian Smith, a 25-year-old fourth year medical student from USC's Keck School of Medicine. We go now to KTLA 5's John Moore, who is on campus with the latest. John, what can you tell us?"

The reporter stood in a hospital hallway, his red tie the sole spot of color against the backdrop of ubiquitous beige-and-white walls and fluorescent lighting.

"According to fellow classmates," the reporter said, "the alarm went out yesterday, when Brian Smith failed to show up for a scheduled weekend shift on his clinical rotation, and did not respond to multiple attempts to contact him. Early this morning, LAPD officers found him in a closet inside his apartment, where he had apparently hanged himself.

"Students and staff are still in shock over the death. The school administration has responded by holding an open forum meeting tonight for members of the medical school community. The Vice President for Student Affairs announced that grief counseling and other resources will be made available to USC students.

"Here with me to talk about today's events is Dr. Lily Reid, a research fellow in healthcare policy at the RAND Corporation, and an advisor to the board of the American Foundation for Suicide Prevention."

Wolf stared as the camera panned left, showing Lily wearing an austere gray suit and somber expression.

"Thank you, John," Lily said. "First off, my heartfelt condolences to Brian Smith's family and friends. I know firsthand how difficult it is to lose a loved one to suicide. Believe me when I tell you that you are not alone. Please do not suffer in silence. Help is just a phone call away. The American Foundation for Suicide Prevention is just one of many organizations that provide counseling and support services. You'll find contact information for local groups at the bottom of this screen, or by going to AFSP.org."

"Dr. Reid," the reporter said, "the administration brought you in today to help organize the school's response to today's tragedy. Can you tell us what USC plans to do?"

"Since I'm here in a purely advisory role," Lily said, "I'll defer that question to Dr. Carry."

A tall man with a shaved head and the body of a linebacker joined them. The caption at the bottom of the screen identified him as Professor Ainsley Carry, Vice President for Student Affairs.

"Our goal at USC," he said, "is to provide students with the best possible education in a safe, healthy, and supportive environment. But sometimes, despite our best efforts, tragedies happen.

"Today we mourn the loss of a promising young man. As we come together to grieve and honor Brian Smith's memory, we must also recognize his passing as a wakeup call. We need to do whatever it takes to prevent a repeat of today's tragedy.

"To this end, we've started mobilizing our local mental health community to ensure that any student or staff member who needs counseling has access to it. This is in addition to our two in-house clinical psychologists who already offer free, confidential counseling to students through our new wellness initiative. And of course we're continuing to develop various programs to help our students with time- and stress-management."

"Thank you, Dr. Carry," the reporter said. "Dr. Reid, anything you'd like to add?"

"We're facing a national crisis," Lily said. "Nearly a million people will lose their physician to suicide this year alone. Why? Because burnout and depression in the medical profession are at an all-time high. And physicians who try to seek help are often stigmatized and face stiff penalties—up to and including the loss of their medical license. We need to eliminate the stigma surrounding mental illness, and tell the doctors who are so busy taking care of us that they must not forget to take care of themselves."

The network went to commercial, and Wolf muted the sound.

The phone rang. He lunged for it, then frowned. Not Lily.

Sighing, he pressed the green icon. "Hi, Mom."

He listened with half an ear as she gave him a run-down on each of his siblings, their wives and children.

"So when are you coming to visit?" she finally said.

He rubbed his eyes. "I don't know. It's been…busy."

"Thanksgiving will be here soon. You'll be here for that, I hope?"

"Wouldn't miss it."

"Any chance you might bring someone with you this time?"

He sighed and glanced at the screen. Another commercial. "It's getting late, Mom—"

"It's barely seven."

"Yeah, but I'm working tomorrow." He turned off the TV. "Listen, Mom, can I borrow the backyard for a day?"

"You're shooting a new video?"

"Yeah."

"The neighbors complained about the noise last time. This isn't another heavy metal piece, is it?"

"More like classic rock," Wolf said. "Very low-key."

"Humph. When are you going to use some decent music for a change?"

"You want me to do a parody video of Handel's *Messiah*?" He waited a few beats. "Yeah, didn't think so."

"Fine. You can use the backyard anytime. As long as it's during reasonable hours, say seven a.m. to seven p.m." She paused. "How many people should I expect?"

"We'll need a lot of bodies for this one. Let me see who I can round up first, okay?"

"Let me know."

"Will do. And Mom? Thanks."

Lily towel dried her hair, pulled on a robe, and padded barefoot to the kitchen.

She'd missed lunch and dinner, and even though the thought of food made her stomach churn, she unearthed a packet of instant oatmeal and put on the kettle.

While waiting for the water to boil, she checked her phone.

A text from Parker: *You OK? Call me.*

He must have caught the coverage. Which meant that some regional or even national affiliate had picked up the story.

Good. She couldn't fight a silent epidemic without the media's help. The more airtime the issue got, the better the chances that something would actually be done about it.

USC's efforts in the wake of the latest suicide were a good start. But Lily had seen other institutions pledge to take action, and as soon as the spotlight shifted away, they reverted to business as usual.

To be fair, there were a handful of medical schools that had already implemented some kind of wellness program. But there were still another hundred and seventy-some schools with nothing in place, and many of them continued to deny that there was even a problem.

The water boiled. She dumped the oatmeal into a heavy mug, stirred in the water, and set it aside to thicken.

For years, Parker had been her rock. Shared grief brought them together, but lately other things superseded that.

Friendship.

Working toward a common goal.

They met and talked regularly, though most of those discussions now revolved around the cases she brought him. Physicians battling discrimination. Wrongful termination suits. Defamation claims. With each victory, they came one step closer to dismantling the wall.

She dialed, and Parker picked up on the second ring.

"You heard?" she said.

"Yes. How are you holdin' up?"

She leaned against the counter. "Fine."

"Do you need me to come up?"

"Not this time. Thanks."

"You sure? Because I can cancel my appointments for tomorrow and be there in a few hours."

"Parker, I'm fine. Seriously. You can't keep rushing up here every time something happens."

He sighed. "If you're sure."

"I'm sure."

"Okay." He paused. "You looked good."

"You're a lovely friend."

"I mean it."

She brought the oatmeal to the kitchen table and sank down in a chair. "Any news on the Wiggs case?"

"Not yet. I'll let you know. You sure you'll be okay?"

"Goodnight, Parker."

"Night, Lil. Call if you need me."

"Thanks." She hung up, then jumped when the phone vibrated in her hand.

Wolf.

Pick up, or let it go to voicemail?

She'd already ignored or brushed off his earlier texts. Her last-minute cancellation of their plans this morning with barely any explanation hadn't gone over well, but at the time she was more concerned with getting Wolf off the phone and responding to the crisis. At the very least, she owed him an apology.

She sighed and pressed the green phone icon. "Hello."

"Lily. Are you home?"

"Yes. Sorry about earlier—"

"I saw you on TV."

She leaned back and closed her eyes. "So you got to experience some of my reality."

When he didn't answer right away, she sighed. Just because she felt raw and beaten didn't mean she had to lash out at Wolf. Besides, she didn't want to reopen that argument. Not tonight.

"I'm sorry," he said. "Can I come over?"

"What, now?" She frowned and glanced at the clock. "It's late. I'm tired."

"We'll just talk," he said. "I promise not to stay long."

"Wolf—"

"I've got some chocolate salted caramel ice cream with your name on it."

She stared at the congealing oatmeal in front of her. "Don't you have to be at work at some ungodly hour in the morning?"

"Not until seven," he said. "So about that ice cream…you want a different flavor? You name it, I'll get it."

For the first time all day, she felt the hint of a smile. "You're bribing me with food again?"

"Whatever works."

"Chocolate salted caramel sounds good."

"Great," he said. "See you in ten."

She answered the door in a long-sleeved gray UCSD T-shirt and baggy sweatpants, her hair in a messy twist, her face devoid of makeup.

If she'd surrounded herself with an electrified fence, the message couldn't have been clearer.

And yet, his body reacted with knee-jerk predictability. As if his subconscious were somehow hard-wired to respond the mere sight of her, the sound of her voice, the clean soap scent of her skin.

He lifted the brown paper bag to eye level. "Ice cream delivery. Chocolate salted caramel, as promised. I even brought spoons."

"Thank you," she said. "Do you want a cup or a bowl?"

He trailed after her. "Tastes better straight from the carton."

"Fine, then you have the carton," she said. "And I'll take a bowl."

"You sure? Because I don't mind sharing. More fun that way."

She stopped abruptly, and he almost ran into her.

"If you're looking for fun," she said, "you might as well turn around and go home."

A month ago, he might have considered it. But then a month ago, he hadn't met Lily.

He reached out and touched her shoulder. "I'm sorry, Lil."

She shrugged.

"You've had a rough day." He stepped in front of her and hesitated. She was looking at the floor, her expression hidden from view. "You said you're tired. Do you want to lie down? I can make you some tea—"

"I don't want tea."

"Okay. You tell me what you want and I'll get it."

She shook her head and wrapped her arms around herself.

"Lil?"

Oh, fuck. Were those tears?

He dropped the bag and pulled her into his chest. Fine tremors shook her frame.

"Shh, it's okay." His lips found her temple.

She remained stiff in his arms. Which was a good thing, considering he'd gone from half-mast to fully erect the moment he'd touched her. Any closer, and she'd peg him as an insensitive sex-obsessed SOB. But as long as she didn't move...

Ah, shit. Her arms loosened. Her hands crept around his waist.

He was fucked.

Back off now, or wait until she pushed him away?

"Wolf?"

He tensed. "Yeah?"

"The ice cream's going to melt."

What the...? She was worried about *ice cream*?

He closed his eyes and breathed out. "Haven't you heard?" he said. "Melted ice cream's the latest rage. Hotter than green smoothies."

She rewarded him with a watery laugh before pulling back and scrubbing her cheeks with her sleeve. "I'll just, um—" She gestured down the hall.

Twenty minutes later, the ice cream was gone and they were sipping chamomile tea that Wolf found in a cabinet while searching for bowls.

Lily sat in the corner of the living room couch, legs tucked beneath her. Wolf sprawled next to her, feet resting on the coffee table.

"Don't worry," he said, catching her look. "I'll disinfect everything before I go. I'm sure you've got a stockpile of Lysol somewhere."

She flushed. "I didn't say anything."

"You didn't need to. You do this thing with your nose, like this—" He demonstrated.

"I do not."

He nodded. "You do."

"Fine," she said. "The Lysol wipes are in the kitchen, beneath the sink."

He set aside his empty mug. "Feeling better?"

"Yes. Thanks."

"Want to talk?"

She took a sip of tea. "Not really."

Wolf leaned back and laced his fingers across his stomach. For several minutes, he studied her in silence.

She'd changed into a fresh shirt, and her color was back. But there was still a pinched look about her lips, and her eyes remained shadowed.

"Did you know him?" Wolf said. "The kid who killed himself?"

She blinked. "No."

"So how'd you get involved?"

She rested the mug on her knee. "I do a lot of crisis management consulting. And I've worked with Ainsley before. A few years ago, when one of the faculty physicians at USC committed suicide."

Wolf vaguely remembered hearing about the death. The man had been the friend-of-a-friend, and several of the doctors from St. Mary's had gone to his memorial service.

He frowned. "That thing you said, about losing someone to suicide. Is it true?"

Her fingers tightened around the mug. "Yes."

"Who was it?"

She shook her head.

Wolf lowered his feet to the floor and moved closer. Easing the cup from her hands, he set it on the table. "Lily." Her fingers felt like ice beneath his. "What happened?"

She stared at their joined hands. "I had no idea he was even depressed."

"Who?"

"Nick," she said. "My fiancé."

A bolt of red hot jealousy shot through him. He tamped it down and managed to keep his voice level. "You were engaged?"

"He was a surgery resident," she said. "Just starting his second year. On call every other night. I mean, who wouldn't be miserable? Technically, it was supposed to be every third night. But no one follows ACGME rules. Especially in surgery. You're told to lie when the Joint Commission comes around. Tell them what they want to hear. *Of course I don't work more than 80 hours a week. Sure, I get to go home after 24 hours of patient care plus four hours to do charts and tie up loose ends.*"

"I'm sorry," Wolf said.

She shook her head and pulled away. Scooting back into the corner of the couch, she pulled her legs into her chest and wrapped her arms around them.

"No one dares tell the truth," she said. "Because then the program would get in trouble, and you'd get slammed with even more work, and on top of that you'd get crap reviews from your attendings—because, let's face it, *you're* the problem here—even though you're busting your butt to take care of more patients than humanly possible and doing your damnedest not let anything slip through the cracks."

Wolf wished he could refute her words. But thinking back to his own residency, he had to admit she was right on the money.

"You want to hear the ironic part?" she said. "I was doing an inpatient psych rotation at the time. Every day I'd go in and see people who were hospitalized for anxiety, depression, suicidal ideation. Every damn day. And at home, when it was staring me in the face, I didn't even recognize it."

"Lily—" He gazed at her, huddled in the corner of the couch, forehead resting against her drawn-up knees. "It wasn't your fault, Lil. You know that. You *know* it wasn't your fault."

She hunched her shoulders. "I had to do something."

And so she did. He saw that now. In a sick way, it made sense. The work she did at RAND. The lectures and workshops. Her involvement with a non-profit focused on suicide prevention.

She'd given up her life as penance for failing to save his.

Jesus, how fucked up was that?

It was her fiancé who'd made the choice. But it was Lily who continued to pay the price. For something that had been beyond her control from the start.

Wolf reached out. Rested a hand on her back before slowly stroking up and down. "Lily."

She rolled her head and looked at him.

"There are physician health committees," he said. "Lots of hospitals have them. Doug chairs the one at St. Mary's."

"I know," she sighed. "But there's an inherent conflict of interest with any physician health committee that's run by a hospital or state medical board. Their priority isn't physician health. It's patient safety."

"Don't you need one in order to have the other?"

"To some extent, yes." She sat up and rolled her shoulders, dislodging Wolf's hand. "But a physician who's struggling with depression or anxiety or alcohol or whatever isn't necessarily impaired. He may just need some help, some extra support. You think that's what the committee provides?"

From her tone, obviously not.

"What the committee sees," she continued, "is a physician who's become a liability. So they conduct an investigation. Call for a hearing. Mandate some officially sanctioned treatment program—most of which are a joke. At best, they're a waste of time and money. At worst, they make the problem worse by threatening punitive action unless the physician agrees to some ridiculous, often arbitrary, requirements. The bottom line is, most physicians would rather suffer in silence than risk going to a physician health committee. And they'll continue to suffer until they either break or quit."

"Look, I know you mean well—" Wolf hesitated as Lily narrowed her eyes. "But maybe quitting's not so bad. There are plenty of things to do besides clinical medicine."

"See, *that's* the problem right there," she said. "That whole macho bullshit mentality that pervades medicine and perpetuates the abuses. Get rid of that, and there wouldn't be any reason to quit."

Christ, were they back to that argument?

Wolf sighed. "I'm sorry about your fiancé, Lil. But he made a choice. That's what it comes down to. He *chose* to take his own life. A different person in the same circumstances might have made a different choice. There are plenty of surgeons who got through residency and have been working in the field for years. Decades. And they're still going. Maybe they're just stronger than your Nick was. More resilient. Better suited to be surgeons. It's not for the faint of heart, that's for sure. But the hours and the pressure are part of the job. That's just the way it is, and no amount of wishing otherwise is going to change that. Maybe you just need to understand and accept that. Deal with it, and move on."

Lily uncoiled herself from the sofa. "That's your advice? Suck it up and move on?"

He eyed her warily. "Well—"

"Fine." She picked up their empty mugs and headed for the kitchen.

Wolf followed. "What are you doing?"

"Moving on," she said. "Maybe you should, too."

"Lil, come on, I was trying to help."

"Well, you've helped enough." She dumped everything in the sink and turned on him. "Thanks for stopping by. We both have an early day tomorrow, so— "

"Lily." He crowded her against the counter. "Baby, don't be that way."

"What way?" She pressed her palms against his chest, preventing him from coming any closer. "I don't know how to be with you. You refuse to listen."

He cupped her face and brushed a thumb down her cheek. "I listen. I just don't always agree."

"*Always*?" She snorted. "How about never?"

"Oh, I don't know." His gaze dropped to her lips. "I think we could come to some kind of agreement tonight."

She sighed and closed her eyes. "I thought you couldn't stay long."

His fingers tangled in her hair and he breathed her in. "I can be persuaded otherwise."

For a moment she hesitated, and then she slid her hands around his neck.

Her lips parted, inviting him in. He growled and took possession of her mouth.

This. This was what he craved. Lily, soft and pliant in his arms, gasping as he lifted her atop the granite counter and stepped between her thighs. The weight of her breasts in his hands, nipples hardening to stiff points as he rolled and pinched them through the thin cotton shirt and lace bra. Her fingers fumbling to unbutton his jeans, tugging the shirt up and the zipper down, fist wrapping around his cock and stroking until he was mindless with need, desperate to be inside her.

"Lily—" He sucked in a breath and caught her wrist. "Pants. Off."

"I'm trying."

"No." He stepped back. "Yours."

Seconds later, she was bare from the waist down, and he was rolling on a condom and plunging into her with a muttered "Sorry" that turned out to be unnecessary because she was already so wet that he slid right in, not quite to the hilt but close enough. Her legs wrapped around his waist, and that was all the encouragement he needed. He gripped her hips and dragged her flush against him, pausing for a moment to catch his breath before pulling back.

"Wolf…"

He drove back into her, again and again, faster, harder, until he couldn't hold off any longer. Burying his face against her neck, he groaned as his release shuddered through him.

He startled awake at two in the morning. For a moment, he lay there, barely breathing, conscious of the warm body nestled against him. His palm rested on the slight curve of her belly, and his cock stirred against the delectable globes of her ass.

Fuck.

He hadn't meant to fall asleep.

And yet he couldn't bring himself to move. Couldn't bring himself to leave her.

He'd have to, of course. If for no other reason than the prosaic need to get to work.

But that was still a few hours away.

And in the meantime, his cock wasn't the only thing stirring.

"Mm," Lily murmured, fitting herself more snugly against him. "What time is it?"

He checked the faint luminous display on his watch again. "Two-ten."

She yawned. "When do you have to leave?"

"You trying to get rid of me again?"

She flashed him a smile over her shoulder. "I have a better idea."

Hell, yeah.

Maybe there was something to be said for staying the night after all.

CHAPTER TEN

Wolf leaned back in his chair and rubbed his eyes. He'd signed out hours ago, but still had charts to finish before heading home.

The flu season was heating up. This week, the hospital census hovered near capacity, while nursing and support staff were stretched to the limit because of so many calling out sick. And the agency temps were next to useless, thanks to some administrator who cited HIPAA concerns as a reason for not granting them temporary access to the hospital's electronic medical record system. The man apparently felt a committee was required to study the situation.

A few more days like this, and Wolf might have to rethink his position on burnout.

Wouldn't Lily be thrilled to hear that?

Speaking of…he'd never gotten around to asking her about the weekend.

His brothers had outdone themselves in recruiting friends to show up as extras for the shoot at his mom's. One more person wouldn't even be noticed. And Lily would get a kick out of participating in the filming process. Especially when she found out the subject of this particular video.

He glanced at the time and winced. Too late to call, but he

could still text. *You awake?*

Working, she responded. *On deadline.*

Wolf's finger hovered over the virtual keyboard. *Can you spare a minute?*

The phone vibrated in his hand. Lily's photo—a shot he'd taken of her aboard the Potomac river cruise—popped up on screen.

He adjusted his Bluetooth headset. "Pizza Hut. How may I help you?"

A moment of silence, and then Lily's voice. "Wolf?"

He laughed. "Yeah. Sorry, I must be hungry. Have you had dinner?"

"It's almost eleven," she sighed. "And I have to get this paper submitted by midnight."

"Sorry. I'll talk fast. We're shooting a video this Sunday in the Valley. Lights, camera, action all day. And food. You in?"

"Sounds like fun," she said. "But I'll be in Seattle. Leaving Friday for three days."

"Oh." He frowned and massaged the throbbing in his temple. "You didn't tell me."

"I just did."

"You're leaving in two days," he said. "If I hadn't called about Sunday—"

"Sorry, Wolf, I don't have time for this. Talk later?"

"Sure," he said. But she'd already hung up.

Damn. Had she just blown him off?

Okay, so she was working on a deadline. He could respect that.

But not telling him that she was planning to be away for the weekend—*again*? Making him drag the information out of her? Weren't couples supposed to share shit like that automatically?

And what the hell kind of relationship did she expect if she was never around?

Whoa. Maybe that was the problem. Maybe she wasn't thinking in terms of relationship.

Was he?

Hell to the fuck no.

He was perfectly happy being on his own.

Except for sex. That he'd prefer to have on a regular basis. Or at least a semi-regular basis. Which was only possible if he and the woman he was having sex with could stay in the same damn city for more than a minute.

A trip here and there was fine. But Lily seemed to be away more than she was actually home.

Maybe he should send her a link to some video conferencing software, so she could conduct business without stepping foot outside her apartment.

Or better yet, phone conferencing software. That way she could put the thing on mute whenever Wolf came by. And while whoever she had on the line continued to natter away, Wolf could strip and fuck Lily so thoroughly that she'd forget all about saving the world.

At least for a little while.

They shot the video as scheduled over the weekend.

Saturday he and Doug recorded the vocals. The result wasn't perfect, but he had enough of a soundtrack to work with to film several takes with the "band" on Sunday. His brothers backed him up on guitar, bass, and drums, while Wolf went all out on keyboard and vocals.

They shot the rest of the footage using a green screen set up in his mom's backyard. There weren't enough white coats and scrubs to go around, so they had to improvise. Luckily, Wolf was good at that.

He staged the remaining scenes on his mother's patio. The meat grinder, set up on a green muslin-draped table. Discarded liquor bottles on a cement floor. Pills raining down in slow motion. A closeup of himself in scrubs and surgeon's cap, slumped against the wall.

By Monday evening, he was bleary-eyed from too much time at the computer—mastering the soundtrack, editing hours of footage down to three minutes, swapping out the green screen for looped clips of hospital hallways and supermarket conveyor belts, then finally syncing up the audio and video.

Before crashing, he texted Lily. *Are you back?*

He fell asleep waiting for her reply.

CHAPTER ELEVEN

Lily wasn't sure what to expect when she showed up at Wolf's house. He'd texted her the address that morning, along with a cryptic message: *I have something to show you. When can you come?*

He lived a half hour north of her, on a quiet residential street in Brentwood. Late afternoon sunlight filtered through the canopy of fig trees overhead.

The house itself was a Spanish-style bungalow that looked like it could use a facelift. Someone had made a half-hearted attempt at trimming the overgrown ficus hedges. Grass and weeds battled for supremacy in the small front yard and sprouted between broken flagstones that formed a path to the door.

He must have been on the lookout, because the door opened before she could ring the bell.

"Great," he smiled. "You made it. Here, let me take your jacket. Are you hungry?"

"No," she said. "I had a late lunch."

She followed him into a brightly-lit living room/dining area dominated on one end by a large flat panel TV mounted above a fireplace, and on the other end by a floor-to-ceiling family tree wall mural.

"How about something to drink?" he said.

"Water would be great, thanks."

He nodded and disappeared through an arched doorway into the kitchen.

Lily moved closer to the mural to examine the framed photos. Formal portraits competed for space with candid shots. There were children with gap-toothed smiles and babies in Anne Geddes type poses. Cap-and-gown shots and wedding portraits.

"Here."

She jumped at the sound of Wolf's voice at her elbow. He held two glasses of ice water, and offered her one.

"Thanks," she said.

He nodded. "I have a sister-in-law who's an artist. She did this as a housewarming gift."

"It's amazing." She leaned in for a closer look at the picture of four boys arrayed on various limbs of an oak tree: one suspended upside down by his knees, another on his stomach, arms and legs hugging the branch, and the two smallest ones sitting like mirror images of each other on opposite sides of the trunk, legs dangling several feet above the ground. "Which one is you?"

"The one hanging upside down, of course."

Her lips quirked. "Of course."

"Seb's the one doing an imitation of a sloth," he continued. "And two jokers who look like they're about to jump are the twins, Freddy and Joe."

She traced the branches as they spread across the wall, the same faces repeating in a series of photos from childhood through adolescence and into adulthood. Smaller shoots branched off, bearing miniature photos of children whose features clearly originated from the same gene pool.

She sighed. "Must be nice, having a big family."

"It's okay," he shrugged. "If you don't mind the noise, and everyone getting into everyone else's business."

She frowned at him. "Better than being ignored."

"I'm not complaining," he said. "I love my mom and

brothers and all their rugrats. But I'm not gonna lie. I like having my own space. Far enough away from all that—" he waved at the wall "—to make sure they can't drop in whenever they feel like it."

She glanced back at the mural. Was he trying to warn her to keep her distance?

Well, he could rest easy. She liked having her own space too. And she wasn't looking to trade it in for a cozy domestic partnership. At least on that score, she and Wolf were in perfect agreement.

"You had something you wanted to show me," she said.

"Yes." He touched her elbow. "Come. I have a studio out back."

She followed him, shivering at the sudden drop in temperature as the wind picked up. They traversed the short distance from the main house to the detached garage. At first glance it looked as dilapidated as the rest of the property. But when he opened the door and flipped on the lights—

"Wow," she said, stopping in the doorway to absorb the setup.

It resembled a control room from some of the cable news shows where she'd made guest appearances. Huge video monitors were arranged in an arc around a central console bristling with dozens of knobs, buttons, and faders. A large triple-paned glass window looked into a second room, which remained dark.

"Here." He offered her a rolling chair, then settled into its twin beside her and dimmed the lights.

One of the screens flared to life, and the faint blip-blip of a heart monitor started up somewhere behind her. She glanced around. "What's that?"

"Surround sound," Wolf said, adjusting the volume.

Images flickered across the screen. A dim hallway, shadows dancing on the wall. Drums, in sync with the heartbeat. The flash of a white coat, stethoscope peeking out from the pocket. A closeup of shuffling feet in surgeon's clogs. Bass, guitar, and keyboards joined in one by one, followed by Wolf's voice:

We don't need your innovation.
We don't need your brain at all.

The camera zoomed out slowly, revealing a long queue of figures wearing blank masks, scrubs and lab coats, trudging down the hall toward a distant door. One by one they stepped through the door and onto a conveyor belt.

The scene cut to a man in a business suit standing on stage, pounding the podium as he sang:

We just need your blind allegiance
To our corporate protocol.
Hey! Doctor! Your work's not done yet.

Behind the man, a huge screen flashed projections of bar graphs with rapidly alternating titles. *Quality Metrics. Press-Ganey Scores.*

Lily glanced at Wolf sitting beside her. His eyes were glued to the monitor, lips moving silently along with the lyrics.

See more patients. Treat and street them. The extra mile?
Not our style. Just do the basics. Oh, yeah—and smile.

She turned back to the video.

The zombie-doctors were back, dropping off the end of the conveyor belt into a massive meat grinder. A quick shot of the businessman hammering his fist on the podium, before the camera cut away to the band performing, with Wolf on keyboards, singing:

We don't care if you're exhausted.
We don't care if you are sick.
You have not fulfilled your quota.
See more patients, make it quick.
Hey! Doctor! Your work's not done yet.

The final sequence returned to a single blank-faced doctor, slumped on a cement floor, his back propped against the wall. Empty liquor bottles littered the floor around him. With shaking fingers, he opened a prescription bottle. Pills spilled out in slow motion.

Can't acknowledge that you're burned out—
Or you might just lose it all.
So you drink and self-prescribe meds
Till you stumble and you fall.

The music faded out, until all that was left was the heart monitor, which beat once, twice, three times, and then flatlined.

Lily sat in silence, staring at the darkened screen.

"Well?" Wolf said. "What do you think?"

She blinked as the recessed lights came back on. "That was…" She blew out a breath. "Wow."

"That's all I get?" He cocked his head. "How about, *'You're amazing, Wolf. You're brilliant. You're my hero.'*"

She smiled. "Thank you, Wolf. Seriously. That *was* amazing. And brilliant. When did you make it?"

"Over the last few weeks." He rolled back his chair and stretched out his legs. "Remember that storyboard I showed you?"

"It was for this?"

"Yes," he nodded. "But the video's not finished."

"What's left?"

"The informational spiel I do at the end. This topic…I just couldn't." He drummed his thumb against the armrest of his chair. "But since you're the expert, maybe you'd like to do it?"

Her mouth fell open. "Really?"

"Really."

She pressed a hand to her stomach. "Oh my God."

"Is that a yes?"

"Yes." She cleared her throat. "Yes, absolutely. When?"

"I'm off the next couple of days. You game?"

She had meetings, and visitors, and—oh, hell. For this, she'd make time. "How long would it take to film?"

He smiled. "Well, you need to write a script first. No more than a minute, so just stick to the highlights. And nothing too dreary. It has to end on a positive note."

Millions of viewers. For that, she'd stand on her head if he asked. "Okay."

"We can do it in a few takes," he said. "An afternoon. I'll do the lighting and camera work."

"I need to rearrange my schedule." She stood up. "And get something on paper—"

Wolf snagged her hand before she could move past him. "How about you do all that tomorrow?"

"But—"

"Tomorrow," he repeated, reeling her in. "I have something more interesting in mind for tonight."

"You do?" Her eyes rounded. "*Oh*."

"Yes." His slow smile made her heart pound. "Ever make love in a studio?"

She licked her dry lips. "No."

"It's private."

She glanced around. "No cameras on?"

"No. But if you want—"

"Oh, no," she shook her head. "Please don't."

He rested a hand on her waist. "Your call."

She cupped his cheek, the day-old bristles rough against her palm. With a thumb, she traced his lips until they parted. His teeth nipped her skin. A wave of heat spread through her, all the way down to her core.

She sucked in a breath. Strange how much she'd missed him while she was away in Seattle. How much she'd missed *this*.

His hands settled on her hips, pulling her closer. Close enough to bury his nose between her breasts. Close enough to slip a hand beneath her shirt and unhook her bra, pulling the straps down to imprison her arms and give him free access to her breasts. Her nipples tightened as he played with them.

"Wait—" she pulled away to remove the shirt and bra. They dropped to the floor.

Wolf reached for her, but she smiled and danced back. "Uh-uh," she said. "Hands on the armrests."

"What?" he blinked.

She wiggled her index finger. "Down."

"But—"

"Down." She watched as he slowly obeyed, his eyes hot, his nostrils flaring. The muscles in his forearms bunched and his fingers tightened around the armrests as she approached.

His gaze dropped to her breasts.

She smiled and stepped between his spread legs. "Don't move."

She flicked open the top button of his shirt.

He groaned. "Lily."

"I mean it." She undid another button. "Stay still."

His jaw clenched.

She continued to work her way down, ever conscious of the burning gaze following her every move. She hesitated for a moment when she got to the straining bulge of his erection.

His fingers twitched, but other than that he remained still.

She sank to her knees, barely registering the discomfort of the hardwood floor. Her attention was too focused on sliding down his zipper and freeing him from the confines of his jeans.

"Lily—"

"Don't move," she said.

He was hot and hard, too thick to get her fingers fully around him. She brushed a thumb over the bulging veins, up to the purple head that was already leaking clear fluid.

"Please—" he said.

Then he fell silent, except for the harsh rasp of his breath as she slowly stroked him up and down, and the guttural groan when she finally wrapped her lips around him.

The following morning, Lily opened her eyes to an unfamiliar bedroom. Cream walls, plantation-style ceiling fan, dark wood furniture, a bed twice the size of hers.

Crap.

She'd meant to leave last night.

But after the studio, Wolf convinced her to join him in the shower, where he'd proceeded to blow her mind.

"Just returning the favor," he'd told her with a grin.

Which apparently wasn't enough, because then he'd insisted on carrying her to bed. Not to rest, of course. Who needed rest, when there were still so many sensory delights to explore?

And explore them they did. He kept her hovering on the brink of orgasm forever. Every time she thought, *Yes, thank God, finally!*—he'd back off. Again and again. Until she was so desperate she'd have promised him whatever he wanted just to get some relief.

Lucky for her, he hadn't requested anything outrageous.

Except—

"Stay," he'd whispered.

She was so exhausted by then, it was easier to agree than to argue.

She wouldn't stay long, she told herself. Just a little while. Maybe take a short nap, then get up, get dressed, and go home.

Sunlight streamed through the open windows, confirming she'd definitely overslept.

In the background, the sound of running water abruptly cut off, galvanizing her into action.

She slipped out of bed, pausing to wrap the top sheet around herself, sarong-style. Every muscle screamed in protest.

Damn. She'd run half-marathons and felt less sore the morning after.

She glanced around.

There were clothes tossed at the foot of the bed, and draped over a nearby chair, and hanging from a hook on the inside of the open closet door. None of them hers.

The bathroom door opened, letting out a cloud of steam.

"Hey, you're up," Wolf said.

She caught a flash of naked torso as he wrapped a towel around his waist. His dark hair stood up in uneven spikes, and he sported yet another day's growth of beard. She flushed, remembering the pleasure-pain of those whiskers between her thighs. That probably accounted for some of her discomfort now.

Droplets of water slid down his neck and chest. She followed their meandering path across his abs, unable to tear her eyes away. The towel tented slightly beneath her fascinated gaze.

Oh, my. Again?

He cleared his throat. "I was about to make breakfast. You eat eggs?"

She blinked. "Uh, sure."

"Now?" His towel slipped, offering a glimpse of the V-line running from hip to groin. "Or later?"

Her eyes jerked up to meet his. "Sorry?"

"Never mind." He grinned and crossed to the bureau. "I'll get some coffee going."

Her eyes slid down of their own accord to his glutes, which flexed with every step.

A drawer opened and closed. The towel dropped and he stepped into a pair of loose pajama bottoms. He turned, grinning when he caught the direction of her gaze.

"Here," he said, offering her a T-shirt. "Something to wear while your clothes are drying. Not that you don't look gorgeous as is, but you might be more comfortable in this."

"Thanks." Her fingers closed over the soft cotton. "Wait—what happened to my clothes?"

"I put them in the wash." He sauntered toward the door. "There are fresh towels and things in the bathroom. Join me in the kitchen when you're ready."

She continued to stare at the door after he left, her brain scrambling to process what just happened.

For a man who'd been so adamant about needing his own space, he was being awfully blasé about her presence here this morning.

Cooking her breakfast? Laundering her clothes? Acting like he was in no hurry to see her go?

How utterly…bizarre.

She shook her head and headed for the bathroom.

He'd left an unopened toothbrush and sample-sized toiletries atop a neatly folded towel on the counter.

Who was this man, and what had he done with the real Wolf?

She frowned at her reflection. Was she was making too much of this? Allowing her own fears to skew her perception?

For all she knew, this morning-after scenario might be his usual M.O. Maybe he had a huge stash of toothbrushes and soaps hidden in some cabinet, ready for deployment whenever he slept with someone new. And maybe the T-shirt he'd given her had graced the bodies of countless other women who came before her.

She shook out the shirt and lifted it against her chest, examining the effect in the mirror. It was long enough to hit her mid-thigh, a light gray emblazoned with distinctive red and blue lettering that read *PENN*. Was that where he'd gone to college?

There was so much she didn't know about him. So much she wanted to learn.

Oh, no. She wasn't going there. Not ever again. Been there, done that, still dealing with the flashbacks.

Sex was about all she could handle. That, and friendship.

He'd mentioned it himself, when they returned from D.C. At the time, she hadn't put it all together, but now it made sense.

Absolutely.

And if the thought of Wolf having sex with other women made her feel a little ill—because, let's face it, friendship was no guarantee of exclusivity, and he was bound to move on sooner or later—well, she'd get over it.

In the meantime, she'd enjoy herself. Keep it light. Not ask too many questions.

She dropped the shirt on the counter, unwound the sheet,

and turned on the water.

CHAPTER TWELVE

"Can I see?" Lily rushed into the studio's control room, skidding to a stop and grabbing Wolf's shoulder to stay upright.

Wolf grinned.

Since dropping the assignment in Lily's lap two days ago, he'd been amazed by her transformation.

Sure, she'd always come across as passionate and dedicated to her work. But the degree of enthusiasm with which she tackled this project was something new. She was almost giddy with excitement, like a kid who'd just discovered Legos.

While Wolf was having second and third thoughts about the grim subject matter, Lily chattered on about incorporating the video into her lectures, and using it as part of a larger campaign during something called National Suicide Prevention Month. Which was apparently in September, ten months away.

"I went a little off script about half-way through." She removed the lav mic from her shirt collar and handed it over. "So we'll probably have to trim some of it, right? Unless you think one of the other takes was better?"

"There's plenty of footage to choose from." He checked that all the files were saved and backed up, then shut down the computer. "Give me twenty-four hours, I'll edit it and we can watch the final version tomorrow."

"Oh."

He got up. "Is that a problem?"

"I have to work."

"So take a day off like you did today." He headed for the set, to shut down and put away the rest of the equipment.

"Tomorrow's no good." She trailed after him, stepping over cables and moving out of the way as he disassembled the boom stand that held the main microphone in place. "I'm hosting visitors from out of town."

"What about after work?" He unplugged the lights and rolled them one by one against the far wall. "We can order Chinese, watch the video, go to bed early…"

"I can't." She bit her lip. "It's the third Thursday of the month. I have dinner with my parents. What about Friday?"

He shook his head and placed the bar stool she'd used for her monologue back in the corner. "I'm on service Friday through Wednesday. And this time of year, things get pretty crazy. I don't know when—or if—I'll be home."

He flipped off the last of the lights and ushered her out through the control room, pausing for a moment to let his eyes adjust to the glare of the afternoon sun.

"Okay," she said. "Then how about next Thursday? You're off?"

"I'm off." He locked the studio door and turned toward the main house. "But it's Thanksgiving. I'll probably be at my mom's all day. You know, doing the family thing."

"Oh." She stumbled on a cracked paving stone, and he caught her, wrapping a hand around her arm.

"Sorry," he said. "I keep meaning to replace those. I just haven't gotten around to it. You okay?"

When she didn't respond, he glanced at her. Her face was white as milk. "Lil?"

She blinked. "I need to go."

"But—"

"I'll text you." She pulled away and headed for the driveway, where she'd parked that morning.

"Wait," Wolf said. "Your bag. It's still inside. You might need it."

"Oh." She stopped and glanced down at her hands, as if just now noticing that they were empty. "Right. Thanks."

She retrieved her bag and sunglasses from the table in the breakfast nook, where she'd left them after earlier.

Wolf watched her jerky movements and frowned. "You sure you're okay to drive?"

"Yes." She hesitated in the doorway. "Thanks for today. For...everything."

He watched her pull out of the driveway and merge with the mid-afternoon mommy-cade of minivans and SUVs ferrying children from school to soccer and tennis and whatever other activities were in vogue these days.

He spent the rest of the day in his studio, editing. As he stared at Lily's animated expression on camera and listened to her voice, he kept circling back to her abrupt departure.

They were in the midst of coordinating schedules when she'd just shut down.

Was it his mention of family that scared her off?

Strange. Especially when just the other day she'd been so fascinated by his family tree.

Maybe he should have invited her to come along.

His mother would certainly be thrilled. She might even stop nagging him about the whole marriage-and-kids thing. Or at least stop shoving so-called eligible females his way.

Then again, Thanksgiving was for family. That's why he'd always balked at bringing a plus-one. It might even give a woman the wrong idea about his intentions.

Besides, Lily probably had plans with her own family.

It was past midnight when Wolf finally shut down the computer.

He could always find another tweak to make, but there came a point in every project where he had to draw the line.

Now all that was left was getting the final okay from Lily.

Not that he really needed it. But if not for her, he doubted he'd ever have tackled the topic. So the video was as much her baby as it was his and Doug's. And it sounded like she was planning to get a whole lot of mileage out of it.

He checked his phone again, as he had throughout the evening.

No new texts.

He debated for several seconds before sending her a message. *Video's done.*

There. Now the ball was in her court.

CHAPTER THIRTEEN

Lily hated third Thursdays.

She'd taken a break from the monthly ritual a few years ago, when she and her father weren't speaking. But eventually, her mother cajoled them both back to the table.

And now, here she was, in the 5700 square foot house above Montana where she'd grown up, sitting at a dining room table that could accommodate twelve but rarely did, picking at some kale and pine nut concoction whose recipe her mother had likely gotten at a ladies' lunch from another health- and beauty-obsessed woman who never cooked.

They'd already exhausted the topics of the latest mass shooting and most recent hurricane. Both disasters were sufficiently far removed from their everyday reality that neither Frederick Reid nor his wife Marian had much interest in discussing them, other than writing the requisite check to the Red Cross and expressing a few words of sympathy.

Rosa, their housekeeper and cook of thirty-plus years, removed their plates and served the next course: grilled cilantro lime chicken with avocado salsa.

"How is Parker?" Lily's mother said. "We haven't seen him in a while."

"He's fine. Busy."

Marian dabbed her lips with a napkin. "Maybe one of these days we can have lunch at the club. Just the four of us?"

Lily paused in the process of picking the onion out of her salsa. "Uh, sure."

"He's such a lovely boy. Don't you think so, Frederick?"

Lily's father grunted and continued to eat.

"I seem to recall he liked skiing," Marian said. "Maybe you should invite him to Aspen for the holiday. Your father and I are flying to Paris next week, so you'd have the house to yourselves."

Lily glanced up. "You're going to Paris for Thanksgiving?"

"Oh, dear, did we forget to tell you? Your father's giving a talk there. And then we're joining Bob and Linda in Budapest—you remember the Murrays, don't you? We're doing a nine-day cruise on the Danube."

"Sounds like fun," Lily managed to choke out.

"Oh, yes," her mother said. "I've always wanted to see Hungary and I know a cruise isn't exactly the same thing as touring the country but…"

Lily tuned her out.

So what if her parents were going away for Thanksgiving? Lily would be fine on her own. She was used to it.

Her mistake was assuming they'd be having Thanksgiving dinner together.

Thirty-four years of ranking near the bottom of her parents' list of priorities, and she still hadn't learned.

Lesson one: never assume.

Lesson two: the only person she could rely on was herself.

But *Thanksgiving*? That seemed especially cruel.

Though she doubted her parents saw it that way. They obviously thought she'd be fine spending time in the mountains, skiing with Parker.

Except Parker wasn't going to be around. He'd left earlier this week for North Carolina, and planned to stay there a couple weeks, catching up with family and friends back home.

For a split second, she considered inviting Wolf. But then she remembered he already had plans for that day.

"…women's club looking for a speaker, and I said I'd ask you. What do you think?"

Lily blinked. "Sorry, Mom, what was the question?"

"Can you do a talk at our January meeting?" Marian said. "Something about mindfulness. That's a big thing these days, isn't it? And it's your area of expertise."

Frederick snorted.

"I don't know, Mom…"

"It doesn't have to be much. Fifteen minutes would be plenty. Kind of an introduction. And maybe you could lead the group through some mindfulness exercises?"

"For God's sake, Marian. Don't encourage her."

"But Frederick—"

"I mean it," he said. "She's wasted enough time on this nonsense—"

"Dad—"

"What?" He turned on Lily. "You think seven years isn't enough? You think throwing away your career will bring him back?"

"Frederick!"

Lily set the fork down beside her barely touched plate and stood up. "Thanks for dinner."

"We're not done here," her father said, rising from the table and tossing aside his napkin.

"Yes, we are."

"Sit down, damn it. I don't care how old you are or how much you think you know. You are still my daughter, and if I tell you to sit down, you will damn well listen."

Lily glanced at her mother, who stood ashen-faced, hand clasping the back of her chair.

"Have fun in Europe, Mom."

"I'm warning you, Lily," her father said. "If you walk out now, you are no longer welcome in this house."

"Frederick!"

Lily hesitated.

"I talked to your old program director at UCSD," her father continued. "He agreed to take you back. *If* you repeat the second half of intern year, starting in January. Under the circumstances, it's the best I could do."

Lily took a deep breath. "Thanks, Dad. But I'm not going back. I have a career. Sorry it's not the one you wanted for me, but I'm happy with it. And if you'd asked me about this before going behind my back, I could have saved you a lot of trouble."

"Lily," her mother said. "Maybe you should consider…"

"No." Lily retrieved her purse from the credenza and headed for the door. "Goodnight."

Her mother's plaintive voice followed her. "But…what about dessert?"

Softly, Lily shut the door and stepped out into the night.

Sunday morning, Parker called her about the Wiggs case. Things were getting close to settlement.

"I'm thinkin' a couple, maybe three weeks," he said.

"Mm-hm."

"Hey, what's wrong?"

"Nothing. I'm still waking up." She smothered a yawn. "It's six-fifteen here."

"Sorry. Late night?"

"Not really." She adjusted the pillow behind her back. "How are your parents?"

"Fine. Daddy's talkin' about retirin'."

She managed a smile. "He's been talking about that for as long as I've known you."

"Yeah." She could hear the grin in his voice. "But this time sounds like he means it."

"And your mom?"

"Busy helpin' my sister with her kids. Jules is actually hostin' this year for us and her in-laws."

"Oh." Lily swallowed. "That's nice."

"You'll be at your parents'?"

"I'm volunteering at the food bank. They need help sorting

and boxing up donated food."

"Don't you do that every year?"

"Yes."

"So that's the first half of the day. What about the rest?"

"I'm keeping it low-key." She could probably get a long run in. Do her nails. Binge-watch *Game of Thrones*. Eat a tub of ice cream. Chocolate salted caramel.

"Low-key? What does that even mean?" He paused. "You're not fixin' to spend Thanksgivin' with that Wolf guy, are you?"

"No." She sat up. "But that reminds me. Your phone call worked."

"What phone call?"

"To Doug Williams. Your old frat brother? They did the video."

"They did?"

"Yes, and it's amazing." This time her smile was genuine. "Exactly what we need. I haven't seen the final version, but maybe after Thanksgiving…"

"That's great, Lil. I'm glad it worked out. Hold on a minute—" There was a brief murmur of voices, then the sound of a shutting door. Seconds later, Parker was back. "That was my momma. She says hi."

"You should have put her on."

"Trust me, darlin', you do not want my momma anywhere near a phone. She can talk water uphill."

"So that's where you got your gift for gab."

"I'm a lawyer, darlin'. Comes with the territory," he said. "But enough about me. You were tellin' me about Thanksgivin'…"

She ran a hand through her tangled hair. "My parents booked a trip to Europe."

"What? Are you shittin' me? They're leavin' you alone on Thanksgivin'? Jesus, Lil. I know they're your parents, but…"

"Please. Don't."

"I'll come back early and we'll spend the day. Go to the food bank, and then do somethin' fun."

"Are you nuts? You've been planning this trip home forever. You can't just up and leave in the middle of it. Your family—"

"Will be fine without me. 'Sides, I've already been here a week, and I'll see them all again at Christmas. You still remember how to ice skate?"

She blinked at the non sequitur. "I guess. I haven't done it in a while…"

"Don't worry," he said. "We'll have fun. Just leave it to me. I can be pretty resourceful, you know."

He wasn't kidding.

He flew in to LAX Wednesday evening, and crashed on her living room sofa.

Thursday morning, after hours of sorting and boxing up a mountain of turkeys, canned cranberry sauce, and pumpkin pie, they had lunch and spent the rest of the day ice skating.

"I didn't even know this was open today." Lily flopped down beside Parker on a picnic bench beside the outdoor rink, watching as a Zamboni resurfaced the ice.

"Typical," Parker said. "You live in a place your entire life without noticin' what's right under your nose. Takes an outsider to point out the magic."

"All right, Mr. Magician, what else do you have up your sleeve?"

"Patience, darlin'." He draped an arm across her shoulders and dropped a kiss on her forehead. "You can't expect me to give away all my tricks at once."

They were the last ones on the ice when the rink closed at ten.

From there, Parker made a short detour to a local 24/7 steakhouse to pick up a meal he'd ordered ahead. That and a couple bottles of wine got them through the rest of the evening.

It was past two in the morning when Lily finally collapsed into bed, grateful for the friendship and alcohol that had gotten her through yet another Thanksgiving.

CHAPTER FOURTEEN

Wolf loped up the stairs to Lily's apartment, to-go box of freshly baked bagels and shmear in hand. He rang the bell, waited twenty seconds, then rang again.

She opened the door wearing an oversized T-shirt and boxers, her hair a glorious mess.

"Wolf?" She winced and pressed a hand to her temple. "What are you doing here?"

He lifted the box. "I brought breakfast."

Okay, so maybe it was presumptuous of him to just show up on her doorstep like this. But he hadn't seen her in over a week, and between her schedule and his, he figured it might be another week before they pinned down a time to watch the completed video. Which was why he'd taken the initiative to bring food and a flash drive without waiting for her response to his early morning text.

"I'm sorry." She leaned against the edge of the door, eyes half-closed. "Did we agree to meet today?"

He'd expected a more enthusiastic welcome. "I texted you this morning…"

"You did?" She pushed the hair out of her eyes and smothered a yawn. "I'm not really awake yet."

"If you let me in, I'll make you some coffee." He dangled

the box in front of her. "And these are still warm."

"Mm." She backed up and opened the door wider. "Give me a few minutes—"

"Hey, darlin'," a man's voice drawled. "You're out of milk."

Wolf stiffened and looked over Lily's shoulder.

A man with blond hair and lanky build wandered out of the kitchen, holding a carton of milk. He wore running shorts and nothing else. Cool gray eyes locked on Wolf.

"Hello." The man straightened to his full height, which put him an inch or two shy of Wolf's own six feet. "Who are you?"

Wolf narrowed his eyes and clenched his fingers into a fist. Instead of answering the question directly, he turned to Lily. "Am I interrupting something?"

"Oh, for God's sake," Lily muttered. "Wolf, meet my friend Parker Atkinson. Parker, this is Wolf Knox. He and Doug made the video I told you about."

Wolf bristled. He should have known. Parker, her *friend*. While Wolf was now demoted to the guy who'd made her video.

"So," Lily said. "Are you coming in?"

Wolf stepped inside. Parker didn't move.

Lily, caught between them, sighed and elbowed Parker in the ribs. "Stop trying to intimidate him." And then she turned to Wolf and frowned. "And you, play nice. I'm going to grab a shower. Five minutes. And I expect you both to behave."

With a final pointed look in Wolf's direction, she swept down the hall. The bathroom door shut behind her.

Five minutes wasn't long. But it was enough to wipe the supercilious smirk off the asshole's face. A quick one-two punch to the gut, another to the jaw, and Lily's friend Parker would be out for the count.

Except that wouldn't solve the problem, would it?

Five weeks ago, she'd told Wolf she that wasn't involved with anyone else. And Wolf believed her.

So what the fuck was Parker doing here now, at eight in the morning, without a goddamn shirt on? And with Lily looking like she'd just rolled out of bed?

The urge to do some damage to pretty boy's face was so strong that Wolf had to move before he gave in to temptation.

Deliberately pushing past Parker, Wolf headed for the kitchen. There were two mugs of coffee on the counter, one with milk, the other black.

Wolf scowled and dumped the bagels on the table.

"There's a Whole Foods two blocks away," he said, turning on the water and reaching for the soap. He didn't bother looking up as Parker crossed the room to throw the empty carton into a pull-out trash bin. "I'm sure they have milk."

"I'm sure they do," Parker said.

Wolf tossed aside the paper towel. "You might want to put on some clothes. It's cold out. And I hear the police are cracking down on public nudity."

Parker's nostrils flared. "Listen up, Wolfman. She wanted your help with her pet project because you're a funny guy. But the project's done, so no need for you to hang around."

Wolf clenched his jaw. "How about we let Lily decide that?"

"Decide what?" Lily stepped into the kitchen. She'd put on a scoop-neck blouse and dark jeans, and slicked her hair back in a low pony-tail.

"Nothin'." Parker pasted on a smile. "Your friend here was just leavin'."

"Actually," Wolf said, "Parker volunteered to do a run to Whole Foods for some milk."

"Oh. Thank you, Parker. If you're sure you don't mind." Lily reached for the box of bagels. "I'll save some of these for you."

Wolf's smile was all teeth. "Of course he doesn't mind."

Parker glowered at him.

Lily glanced up. "Parker?"

For a moment, Wolf thought the man would balk. In Parker's place, Wolf would have flat out refused to leave. Allow a rival to stay behind with Lily? Alone? *Hell, no.*

But Parker surprised him. Instead of digging in his heels, he shot Wolf a final glare, then turned to face Lily. His expression softened.

"You got it, darlin'," he said.

Wolf watched as the man headed for the living room, where he retrieved some clothes from a suitcase that Wolf hadn't noticed until now. A minute later, he emerged from the bathroom, fully dressed.

Lily walked him out.

Wolf moved closer, but their voices were too low for him to distinguish the words.

The door closed, and Lily returned to the kitchen to find Wolf hanging his jacket on the back of a kitchen chair.

"Well?" She crossed her arms over her chest. "Care to tell me what that was about?"

Wolf clenched his jaw. "He spent the night."

"Two nights," she said. "On the fold-out sofa. He flew in for Thanksgiving. So what?"

The tightness in Wolf's chest eased a little. "You didn't sleep with him."

"Of course not," she said. "And I thought we already had this conversation."

"We did. Sorry." He rubbed the back of his neck. "What about your parents?"

"They're in Europe."

His fingers stilled at her clipped tone. Was that impatience in her voice? Anger? Something else?

He studied her.

A hint of vulnerability shimmered in her eyes before she lowered her lashes.

"If you wanted some company," he said slowly, "you could have called me."

"You were with your family."

"And Parker wasn't?"

She shrugged. "They understood why he needed to leave."

"Then explain it to me," Wolf said. "Because I'm totally in the dark here."

She leaned against the wall and closed her eyes. For several moments she simply stood there, not moving, barely breathing.

Wolf's gut tightened.

And then she began to speak, so softly that he had to lean forward to catch the words.

"Thanksgiving was when it happened," she said. "I was on call the night before. I signed out that morning and came home and found Nick…"

"Jesus." Wolf reached her in two strides, then hesitated. Her eyes were still closed, and she looked paler than the wall behind her. *Ah, fuck it.* He wrapped her in his arms. "I'm sorry, Lil. Why didn't you tell me?"

"Parker came," she said, her voice muffled against Wolf's shirt. "He was Nick's best friend. He got there right after the paramedics. If not for him…" She let out a long, shuddering breath. "He helped me get through it. We helped each other."

"I see." Wolf buried his nose in Lily's hair, breathing in the familiar scent of berries.

In her eyes, Parker was a friend. A close, trusted, *platonic* friend. Not a lover.

Wolf was the man she'd welcomed into her bed.

But that didn't mean Parker was happy with the arrangement. Or that he'd let it stand in perpetuity. When Lily walked into the room, the naked emotion that transformed Parker's face was painful to watch. The man was in love, no question about it.

What could Wolf offer Lily to compete with that?

Parker returned with the milk, and the morning deteriorated from there. Both men growled and sniped at each other like dogs circling the same bone.

Wolf, she wasn't surprised. Volatility and sarcasm were as much a part of his persona as his uncompromising work ethic and his love for music.

Parker, though? What the hell was wrong with him? She knew he was protective of her, and had been ever since Nick died, but this surliness was something she'd never seen from him before. Even when she'd watched him in court, he was the consummate Southern gentleman—almost a caricature of the real thing—but it worked. Judges and juries loved him.

It turned out Wolf brought not just bagels but also a thumb drive with the final video on it. They watched it on her computer, sitting on the floor in front of the coffee table, Lily in the middle, their backs propped against the sofa.

Parker jostled her shoulder. "One of these days, darlin', you're goin' to have to splurge on some real furniture."

"This *is* real furniture," she countered.

Wolf shushed them both and pressed play.

For nearly four minutes they watched in spellbound silence. Even Parker seemed at a loss for words.

After the screen faded to black, he shook his head and muttered something about fifty million Elvis fans.

Wolf stood and offered Lily a hand up. "So do I have the green light to post it?"

"Yes," she said. "Thank you."

He nodded. "I'll send you the link tonight. Keep the thumb drive."

"You're okay with me using it for talks and workshops?"

"It's yours," Wolf said.

Parker cleared his throat. "I'm starvin'. There's a place on Colorado that does elk burgers with crispy onion, cheddar, BBQ sauce, and homemade tater tots on the side. How about it, Lil?"

Wolf jumped in before Lily could answer. "We just had breakfast."

Parker curled his lip. "That wasn't breakfast. That was an appetizer."

"How about this," Lily said. "Parker, I'll make you a sandwich to go. And Wolf, thanks for stopping by and...everything. I'll walk you down to your car."

"You're kicking me out *again*?" Wolf groused.

"I've got work to do," she said. "There are big-wigs coming to RAND next week, and I have a presentation to prepare for them that I haven't even started. So yes, I'm kicking you *both* out."

While Parker packed his suitcase, she walked Wolf to the parking lot.

"Come here," he said, leaning back against his car.

He drew her flush against his body and framed her face with his palms. Their kiss started out slow, melting her by degrees, until she was pliant as warm taffy in his hands.

"Come home with me," he murmured.

His hands settled on her hips. She could feel him hard against her. For a moment she wished she could just give in, toss aside her responsibilities, and indulge in an afternoon of pure physical pleasure. But that would put her even farther behind, and she hated the anxiety that came with scrambling to catch up.

She sighed. "I can't. I really do have work…"

"This weekend, then."

She kissed his chin, the corner of his mouth, and then forced herself to step away. "I'll call you."

CHAPTER FIFTEEN

He'd used the words often enough himself to know they meant nothing.

I'll call you was not a statement of intent, or a reflection on how well or poorly the date had gone. The phrase was nothing but a polite punctuation mark, letting both parties know that the evening was over. Which left things as open-ended as possible, without hurting anyone's feelings.

The problem was that sonofabitch Parker was still in her apartment when Wolf left. Who knew what damage the man could wreak in Wolf's absence?

Wolf held off texting Lily till this morning.

She replied with an emoji of a woman behind a computer, followed by the two words he was beginning to hate: *Still working.*

His response—*Break for lunch?*—was met with silence.

Now, sitting on Doug and Tina's living room couch while Doug closed the snaps on his son's onesie, Wolf fiddled with his cell.

Text her again?

Call?

Bypass the whole phone thing altogether and just show up with food?

He opened the YouTube app and checked the stats. Over a hundred thousand hits. Not bad for a video posted just yesterday.

The comments were mixed. From *Nice job* and *Amen!* to *What a drag* and *Stop whining, you're still in the 1%.*

There were even a few comments that he promptly deleted. He didn't know if *BigDick* from Montana was trying for irony, but Wolf certainly didn't want Lily seeing *Shut up and bend over.* And what kind of cretin watched a video about physician burnout and wrote *I wanna fuck that b*tch?*

What was wrong with people these days?

Maybe he should just disable comments on the video completely. Or change the settings to allow inappropriate comments to be filtered and held for review. Yeah, that sounded like a plan.

He scrolled to the settings and quickly made the changes, then resumed reading.

Doug's voice interrupted. "Don't get me wrong, bro. I enjoy your company. But mind telling me why you're here again?"

Wolf scowled. "My bike's still in the shop. And there's a high surf advisory in effect through tomorrow."

"So you decided to come and hang out with me and Isaac?"

"It's my birthday." Wolf shrugged. "I didn't want to drink by myself."

"Oh, that's right. Happy birthday, bro." Doug eyed Wolf's barely touched bottle on the coffee table. "Doesn't look like much of a celebration, though."

"The rest of the beer's in the fridge," Wolf said. "Help yourself."

"Thanks." Doug cocked his head. "You don't look too happy."

"I'm saving that for tomorrow. My mom's having the family over."

"Ah. Well, I'm sure that'll be fun." Doug scratched his ear. "Listen, I'm sorry to have to break this party up, but Isaac and I need to go for a walk. It's the only way he'll take an afternoon nap. You're welcome to join."

Damn. Had it really come to this? Wolf and Doug, until recently active subscribers to the work-hard-and-party-harder approach to life, strolling the streets of Santa Monica on a Saturday afternoon, diaper bag strapped to Wolf's back, and infant in a Baby Bjorn adorning Doug's chest.

Wolf's brothers would bust a gut laughing if they could see him now.

Ten minutes into the stroll, Wolf broke the silence. "How well do you know Parker?"

"Who?"

"Parker Atkinson. Your fraternity brother."

Doug shrugged. "Frankly, until he called a few weeks ago about doing the video, I'd forgotten all about him. He was a few years behind me in college. I graduated, moved up to L.A. for med school. He apparently stayed in San Diego and went to law school. Last time I saw him was about six, seven years ago. I was fresh out of fellowship. Just joined St. Mary's. I was dating—what was her name? Tall, with killer legs and tits out to here—"

"That," Wolf said, "would describe most of the women you dated before Tina."

Doug grinned. "Yeah, well. Can't say I miss it. Tina's one in a million."

"A paragon among women," Wolf said, straight-faced.

"Don't mock it till you've experienced it, bro. Love has a way of knocking you flat on your ass, and whatever you thought was important before? Completely irrelevant. Whole different set of priorities."

Wolf frowned. Was that what was happening here? Were his priorities undergoing a sea change thanks to an opinionated, slightly OCD, workaholic female with a quick wit and quicker tongue?

True, she challenged him at every turn and made him question long-held beliefs. And in her presence, he felt more alive and engaged than he had in...longer than he cared to admit.

But was that love?

He stepped off the curb, only to be jerked back as a car whizzed by.

"Are you fucking insane?" Doug said. "That was a red light."

Whether from the sudden movement or from his father's raised voice, Isaac woke up and started crying.

"Shh, it's okay," Doug murmured, cradling the baby's head and swaying from side to side. "Your uncle Wolf just forgot to look both ways while being his usual idiot self and trying to cross on a red light."

"Thanks," Wolf said, shaking off his bemusement. "But would you mind skipping the insults?"

"Just making sure Isaac understands what *not* to emulate."

"Right." The kid stopped crying just as the light changed. Wolf made a show of looking both ways before crossing. Once they were all safely on the other side, he redirected the conversation back to the original topic. "About Parker…?"

"Oh. Right." Doug adjusted the cap on Isaac's head. "So I promised this girl a week up at Lake Arrowhead, and we ended up cutting it short to drive down to San Diego for the funeral. Nick, the guy who died, was a frat brother. So most of our frat house turned out, including Parker. Anyway, that's the last time I saw him, or had any contact with him until he called out of the blue with an idea for a video."

"That's it?"

"Yes," Doug said. "Why do you ask?"

Wolf readjusted the shoulder straps of the diaper bag. "I was just wondering if you knew what the deal was with him and Lily."

"Lily who?"

"Fuck. I thought mommy brain only happened to women." Wolf blew out a breath. "Lily Reid. You know, the woman you invited to talk at the Post-Graduate Assembly? The one who did the PSA at the end of our video? *That* Lily Reid."

Doug raised his brows. "My hearing is perfectly fine."

"Good." Wolf lowered his voice. "But your memory could

use a tune-up."

"It's all about context, bro. Of course I know who Lily is. I'm sorry I missed her talk at the Assembly. She did a workshop last year on finding meaning in medicine. Powerful stuff. That's actually what got me thinking about setting up this year's program, and inviting her to be keynote speaker." He paused to look at Wolf. "So she and Parker are an item?"

"Hell, no." Even hearing Doug say the words made Wolf see red. "They are *not* an *item*."

"Well, no need to jump down my throat. You're the one who brought it up."

Wolf gritted his teeth. "You don't remember meeting Lily at the funeral?"

"You mean Nick's funeral?" Doug scratched his jaw. "No, but I guess it's possible. There were a lot of people there besides the frat brothers. Nick was a popular guy. Played water polo in college, so a bunch of his teammates showed up. Classmates from med school. Residents from his program. He was doing surgery, I think. Dozens of people I assumed were family or friends. And you say Lily was there?"

"She was Nick's fiancée," Wolf ground out. "And Parker was apparently his best friend."

"Get outta here. Really?"

"Really."

"Small world." Doug shook his head. "An experience like that. Christ. No wonder she's so single-minded about fixing the system. And Parker...whoa, hold on. You think she put him up to calling me?"

"I know she did."

"You do?" Doug said. "But why? She could have called me herself. I would have said yes in a minute."

Wolf sighed. "*You* would have. But I'd already turned her down."

"You?" Doug stopped in the middle of the street and stared at him. "What the fuck? *You* turned *her* down?"

"About the video, you moron."

"Oh." Doug furrowed his brow. "But we ended up making

it anyway."

Wolf glanced at his watch. "Would you look at that? Almost five. Time to head back."

"Wait a minute," Doug said. "You did it. That's what this is all about. You hooked up with her after all. After telling me it didn't work out. You *dawg*."

"Keep it down, would you?" Wolf said. "There are children here."

"So…was she any good?"

"For Christ's sake. You're married to Tina, Ms. One-in-a-Million. Get your fucking mind out of the gutter."

"Ooh, touchy. What happened?"

Wolf scowled. "Nothing."

"Something must have, or you wouldn't be so pissed off."

"I'm not—" Wolf broke off. "Fine. You want to know what happened? Parker. *That's* what happened."

"Okay…"

"The guy's a snake. Has Lily totally bamboozled. And now she won't even answer my texts."

"In other words," Doug said, "she's moved on and you're jealous?"

"I'm not jealous," Wolf said. Jealous was too tepid a word for what he was feeling. "The guy's an asshole, that's all."

"Why? Because he's got what you want?" Doug said, as Wolf started to move away. "Wait, where are you going? You can't leave me without a diaper bag!"

Wolf removed the backpack. "Here you go."

Doug shook his head and held up his hands in a sign of surrender. "I'm sorry, okay? If it's that important to you, I'll shut up."

Wolf glared at him for the space of a minute, then nodded and slid his arms back through the shoulder straps.

They walked without speaking for several blocks.

Doug kept casting him worried looks. Finally, he said, "You okay?"

"Yeah," Wolf said. "I just need to get rid of Parker."

"Get rid of him, how?"

"Oh, I dunno. Drug him and dump his body in the ocean?"

"Ah. Well, not to be a wet blanket or anything…but as your best friend, I feel it's my duty to point out you might lose your medical license for doing that. Maybe even go to jail."

"Yeah, well no plan is perfect." Wolf rolled his shoulders to work the kinks out. "I just need more time with Lily. Show her that what I can offer her is exactly what she needs and wants."

"Do you even know what that is?"

Wolf opened his mouth, then closed it without answering.

What did Lily want?

Well, there was the obvious. The cause that sucked up so much of her time and attention: reforming the pressure cooker culture of medicine and graduate medical education on a system-wide level.

But what did she want for *herself?*

Money? Considering her background, she was probably all set there.

Someone to take care of her? Ha. Aside from his mother, he'd never met a more independent, self-sufficient woman.

And then it hit him. How Lily hung on his every word when he described his brothers. Her wistful expression on seeing the photos crowding his living room wall. The way she'd flinched and quickly changed the subject at his casual, almost knee-jerk response about liking his own space.

Must be nice, having a big family.

He took it for granted. The one thing he had that she coveted.

Wolf smiled and slung an arm across Doug's shoulders.

"Doug, my man," he said, "you're a genius."

CHAPTER SIXTEEN

Lily shut down her computer and stretched.

She hated the busywork involved in drumming up money. But PowerPoint presentations with glitzy animations and dumbed-down language kept the moneybags happy. And they in turn continued to fund her research.

At least she'd knocked this one out in less time than anticipated, leaving her with all of Sunday free.

Her stomach rumbled, and she glanced at the clock. Nine-thirty. No wonder. She'd grabbed a left-over bagel for lunch, but that was hours and hours ago.

A quick glance in the fridge confirmed that nothing new or edible had appeared there since the last time she'd checked. Lean Cuisine it was.

She texted Wolf while waiting for the frozen dinner to heat.

Seconds later, the phone rang.

"Are you busy tomorrow?" he said.

"Not really. Why?"

"My mom's having a party."

"Mm-hm." The microwave pinged. "What's the occasion?"

"My birthday."

"Oh, I didn't know. Happy birthday. Is it a milestone year?"

"Thirty-nine," he said. "So technically, no. But according to my mom, every year's a milestone year. And every birthday and holiday is an excuse to throw a party. There's always a big spread, plenty of food."

She slid the plastic tray onto a plate. "Sounds great."

"I'll pick you up at three."

"Wait a minute—"

"You can't back out now. I already told my mom you'd be there."

"What the…" She nearly dropped the plate on the way to the table. "Why would you do that? What if I already had plans?"

"Do you?"

"Well, no." She sank into a chair.

"Then I don't see the problem. Oh, and wear something you can run in. That you wouldn't mind getting dirty."

"What?"

"We usually have a pick-up football game in the yard before dinner."

"Football?" She propped an elbow on the table and rested her forehead on her upturned palm. "I don't play football."

"That's okay," he said. "You know the rules?"

"Sort of."

"You'll be fine, Lil. It's all in good fun."

"Wait…what did you tell your mom about me…us?"

"That I asked you to marry me but you said no."

"*What?*"

"Kidding," he said. "Relax. You're a friend. It's my birthday. I can bring who I want."

The football game was fun, and luckily no one got hurt—though there were a few close calls.

Wolf's mother, Martha, sidled up to Lily toward the end of the game, by which time Lily and two of the wives had dropped out—one to breastfeed, and the other to help Martha in the kitchen.

"That's the nice thing about having two doctors and a nurse in the family," Martha said. Wolf's older brother Sebastien had apparently gone into family medicine and married a nurse. "Your sons can make idiots of themselves and you don't have to worry about going to the emergency room."

Lily glanced at her. "Did you spend a lot of time in the ER when they were growing up?"

"Oh, you better believe it." Martha shook her head and watched as Wolf plowed into one of the twins, sending them both to the ground in a tangle of limbs. Wolf scrambled up and offered a hand to his brother. "I was on a first-name basis with every nurse in our local ER. I swear, there wasn't a tree in the neighborhood those boys didn't climb. They raced their bikes downhill in the middle of the street—no helmets, of course, no matter how many times I threatened to take away their bikes if they didn't put the damn things on. And then there was the summer they all took turns jumping from the roof of the garage, pretending to be Spiderman. Until Fred finally broke his arm, which put a stop to that."

Lily stared at her. "It's a wonder any of them made it to adulthood."

Martha laughed. "Kids are resilient. You'll see that when you have your own."

"Oh, no—" Lily stepped back. "I'm not having kids."

Martha cocked her head. "Why not?"

"Because…" Lily frowned. How did she even get into this conversation? And with Wolf's mother, of all people! "I'm sorry, Mrs. Knox, but I really don't see how that's relevant here."

Martha studied her for several seconds before nodding and turning back to the game. "You're right. None of my business. But you might want to discuss it with Wolf before either of you gets too much older. He's thirty-nine now, and you're…?"

"Thirty-four." She gritted her teeth and tucked a stray strand of hair behind her ear. "Look, Mrs. Knox, I'm not sure what Wolf told you, but we're just friends."

"If you say so, hon. But you're the first *friend* he's brought home to meet the family."

Lily swallowed and glanced toward the field, where Wolf was at the moment barreling toward the goal.

"Touchdown!" Martha shouted, clapping her hands. "Okay, boys, time to wrap it up. Food's ready."

Laughter and several groans accompanied her announcement.

"Five minutes," Martha called out over the noise. She smiled at Lily. "See you inside."

Wolf tossed the ball to one of his nephews, and trotted toward the sidelines, where he picked Lily up and twirled her around before planting a theatrical kiss on her lips. Catcalls and more laughter rang out.

"Put me down," she said, smacking him on the shoulder. "You're covered in mud. And everyone's staring."

"We can shower it off." He lowered her to the ground, but kept hold of her hand, pulling her toward the house. "Come on, I'll show you where the bathroom is."

"*Now?*"

"Just to wash our hands," he laughed. "Trust me, when I get you into the shower, it won't be where a bunch of jokers can line up outside the door and bang on it, yelling for us to hurry up."

Dinner itself was chaotic. A half dozen conversations going on all at once, laughter and teasing and the occasional sharp admonition directed at one of the kids to *Stop hitting your brother!* or *Sit down.*

By the time Martha brought out a massive sheet cake with chocolate frosting and two lit candles in the form of the numbers three and nine, Lily had relaxed enough to join in with the family's lively rendition of "Happy Birthday."

One of the twins—Joe?—stood up at that point and tapped a fork on his glass. "Attention, please. Before we get to the gift opening part of our program, Freddy and I would like to sing a song we wrote in honor of the occasion. We call it 'Big Bad Wolf.'"

Wolf groaned. "Come on, guys, I'm trying to make a good

impression here."

"Don't worry." Joe winked at Lily. "We saved the embarrassing bits for next year. Ready, Freddy?"

Fred joined his twin at the head of the table. "On the count of three…"

Here's the story of a boy named Wolfgang
Who had big dreams of rappin' like Snoop Dogg.
The only problem with that dream, bro:
His voice made him sound like a bullfrog.

But his mom said, "Wolfie, don't you worry.
There are other things that you can learn to do."
So Wolf studied, and then applied to med school —
Cuz truth is homeboy suffered a loose screw.

Then one day Wolf said, "Yo, what was I thinking?
Giving up my dream without a fight?
I can lip sync, and still be called a doctor —
Chicks dig MDs who can time it right."

Laughter rippled across the table. Joe waved his arms in the air. "All together now, don't be shy."

That's the way he became the big bad Wolf.
The big bad Wolf. The big bad Wolf.
That's the way he became the big bad Wolf.

As several voices joined in on a repeat of the refrain, Lily glanced at Wolf.

He caught her eye and shrugged. "Brothers." As if that one word explained it all.

She reached for his hand beneath the table. Wolf smiled and twined their fingers together.

Fred picked up the melody, reclaiming her attention.

So listen to this lesson, little piglets:

Talent isn't really where it's at.
All you need is super-sized cojones
Like our big bad Wolfman. Yo, you copy dat?

The big bad Wolf. The big bad Wolf.
That's the way he became the big bad Wolf.

One of the children piped up, "What's cojones?"—only to be shushed by his mother, while Fred and Joe ended the song with a rousing flourish.

That's the way—
Oh, yes, that's the way
He became
The Big. Bad. Wolf.

Lily withdrew her hand to join in the applause.

The twins grinned and bowed.

"Now," Wolf's mother said, rising from the table. "Time to open the presents."

Traffic was light on the drive back.

"Doing okay?" Wolf said.

"Fine." Lily kept her eyes closed and concentrated on the soothing strains of Chopin flowing from the car's speakers. "Your family is lovely. Thanks for inviting me."

"My pleasure." He paused. "They liked you too."

She let that go without comment, and they lapsed into silence. The smooth movement of the car, combined with the soft music, lulled her to sleep, and she didn't wake up until they pulled into her apartment complex.

"Nice nap?" Wolf said.

"Mm. It's been a long week. Are you coming up?"

"Sure. If you don't mind me tracking dirt inside."

"I'm dirty too," she said. "And you mentioned something

about a shower…"

That prompted him to move, and she laughed as they raced up the stairs.

"No fair," she said, as he passed her on the second flight, taking three steps at a time. "Your legs are longer."

"You know what they say…" He slowed down and flashed her a grin.

"What?"

He waited until she was level with him before sweeping her up and over his shoulder. "To the victor go the spoils."

"Wolf—!" She grabbed the back of his jacket as blood rushed to her head. For a moment all she could do was blink away the black spots in her vision. And then she focused on a more interesting sight: his tight glutes, flexing with each step.

The temptation to touch was too strong to resist. But before she could get too carried away, he bent forward and set her back on her feet in front of her door.

Somehow she managed to get it unlocked. And then they were inside, and it didn't matter where their mud-splattered, grass-stained clothes landed. All she cared about was his mouth on hers and the feel of his naked skin beneath her questing fingers.

He was the one who slowed things down—enough to get them into the shower beneath the hot spray, where he explored her body, his hands slick with citrus-scented body wash.

"Turn around," he said. "Put your hands on the wall."

He kneaded the muscles of her back, working his way down and around to the front, gliding up her stomach and cupping her breasts, fingers pinching her nipples until she moaned and pressed back against him.

He was hard and throbbing at the small of her back. "Spread your legs."

She did, and closed her eyes as his hand found her inner thigh and slid up, slowly, to her core, where he teased her folds apart and circled her clit with his thumb.

She dropped her head back against his shoulder. "Please."

A finger eased inside her, then retreated. "Please what?"

"I need…"

"What?" His lips moved against her neck, just below her ear. A second finger joined the first, deeper this time, while his thumb continued to tease her clit. "What do you need?"

His fingers kept moving, ratcheting up the tension, until her thighs were quivering and she couldn't think, let alone speak, and then his fingers were gone, only to be replaced by something thicker, while his hands gripped her hips and he drove into her from behind, the force of his thrust ricocheting through her.

"Fuck—" He pulled out, despite her protest. "Turn around."

"What?" She blinked and tried to make out his features in the roiling steam. "Why?"

"No condom." He pressed her back against the wall, and she shivered. The shock of cold tiles at her back soon dissipated beneath the hot water and even hotter male vying for her attention. He claimed her mouth, tongue dueling with hers, chest pressing against her breasts, cock throbbing against her belly.

Blindly, she reached down and wrapped her fist around him, stroking him a few times, until he caught her wrist and pulled her hand back up to his shoulder. "No."

"Why not?"

His lips brushed her ear. "I'm not ready to cum yet."

She wanted to smack him. "Well, I am."

She felt his smile against her neck. "No you're not." He licked the pulse fluttering at the base of her neck. "But you will be. Soon."

He continued down to her breast, tongue swirling around the nipple before sucking hard, while his fingers played with her other nipple, each tug sending a corresponding zing down to her core.

Damn him and his control. She wrapped a leg around his hip and rubbed herself against him. Screw the condom. She wanted him inside her. Skin on skin. *Now*. Wanted him pounding into her until neither of them could stand.

"Wolf…"

He jerked against her, cursed, and then lifted her leg higher, draping it over his shoulder as he knelt in front of her, mouth settling over her, tongue plunging inside, one hand cupping her ass to keep her from edging away, while the other delved into her folds, homing in on the tiny bundle of nerves at the apex, until she was shaking and sobbing his name, and then he pinched her clit and she came so hard she saw stars.

CHAPTER SEVENTEEN

For the rest of the week, Lily rode a post-orgasmic high, topped up every evening when Wolf showed up at her door with food and fresh stories about his brothers and their assorted offspring.

He wasn't due back at the hospital until Saturday, so there was no reason for him to rush home. At least that's what he told Lily, and she didn't question it. There was still the novelty of waking up in his arms, which she wasn't ready to give up just yet. And surprisingly, his continued presence both in her apartment and her life didn't make her feel claustrophobic.

Though there were times when she had to take a deep breath and count to ten or twenty or fifty, to stay calm in the face of his provocative humor.

"Do you even know how offensive that is?" she said, when the counting didn't help.

"Sorry," he grinned. "Just making sure you were listening."

Charming and infuriating, all in the space of a minute.

He was like her own personal improv comedian, doing running commentary on absolutely everything. Entertaining, but also exhausting.

And yet, when he wasn't there, the apartment felt cold and empty and way too quiet. Funny how she'd never noticed that before.

"Don't you get bored, doing the same route every time?" Wolf said, after joining her for the third day in a row on her morning run.

"I do longer runs on weekends," she said. "And a different route when I travel. Obviously."

"Obviously," he nodded. "But the rest of the time it's the same five-mile loop?"

"I like it," she said. "I don't have to pay attention to where I'm going. So I can think about other things. Or just clear my head."

It was still dark out, and the only people they encountered were fellow exercise enthusiasts, dog owners taking their pets for a walk, and a homeless woman wheeling a tarp-covered cart and muttering to herself.

Lily barely paused before breezing through a red light, Wolf at her heels.

"Maybe you *should* pay attention to where you're going," he huffed.

She turned to jog backwards for a few steps. "There aren't any cars out this early."

"What do you call that?" he said, pointing to a car that sped past them.

"An aberration," she said. "And you're just being contrary. You know, you didn't have to get up early just to go running with me."

"One of these days," he said, "I'll teach you how to surf. Now there's something worth waking up early for."

She made a noncommittal sound and picked up her pace.

It was easy to ignore a throwaway comment about some hypothetical future surfing lesson.

But she couldn't ignore a direct challenge. Especially when it concerned her work.

"You're doing *what?*" Wolf said Friday night, over dinner at a nearby sushi place.

She finished her plum wine. "Driving down to San Diego tomorrow to work with Parker. I told you, I have a new case."

"The pregnant urology resident," he said.

"It's a clear case of sexual discrimination," Lily said. "A woman shouldn't have to decide between keeping her pregnancy or her career. The program director was way out of line, and the fact that he blocked her from sitting for the boards on the basis of some trumped-up charge of unprofessional behavior—"

"I get it," Wolf said. "The guy's a jerk. He should be strung up by his thumbs and forced to listen to Gloria Steinem on endless repeat."

"This isn't a joke."

"I know. I'm sorry." He signaled their waiter for the bill. "But it's also not *your* problem. Let the woman get a lawyer on her own. I'm sure there are plenty out there besides your friend Parker who would love to take her case."

"Maybe, but Parker has a lot of experience with this kind of litigation, and he's willing to do it on contingency."

"More power to him. But I still don't see why you have to be involved."

She sighed. "Because I'm the one she reached out to. The least I can do is facilitate a meeting between her and Parker."

A muscle in his jaw jumped. "And that requires you to drive down there tomorrow and sit in on this meeting. In person."

"The woman's thirty-two weeks pregnant, on bedrest. We're meeting at her house. So, yes. I need to be there tomorrow in person."

She pulled on her jacket while Wolf paid the bill.

Outside, the wind whipped her hair into her eyes. She gathered it in a twist and fumbled in her bag for a clip.

Wolf stepped around her, his broad back blocking the worst of the wind.

"Thanks." She let go of her hair and continued to search her purse.

For a minute, he simply stood and watched. Then he reached into his jeans pocket and pulled out an elastic band. "Here."

She glanced up and blinked. "How...?"

"You left it at my place last time."

Last time...as in two weeks ago?

He'd been carrying the thing around in his pocket for *two weeks*, just waiting for the right opportunity to return it?

Yeah, and she was in line to become the next leader of the free world.

More likely, Wolf just happened to see the hair tie tonight on his way out the door, and snagged it along with his wallet and keys.

She reached for the elastic. "Thanks."

He waited while she finger-combed her hair into submission and secured it in a low ponytail, then offered her his elbow.

It was a five minute walk to her place. They completed it in silence.

"Coffee?" she said.

He shook his head. "I'll walk you up, but I can't stay. I'm back on service tomorrow."

At her door, he hesitated. "Lily..."

"Change your mind?"

"No."

She opened the door wider. "You might as well come in and just say it. Whatever you're thinking."

"It's about Parker."

She stiffened. "What about him?"

"The thing is..." He sighed. "Maybe I'll have that coffee after all."

Wolf leaned against the counter, watching her make the coffee.

If only he didn't have to work tomorrow, he could drive down to San Diego with her.

But that wouldn't solve the problem. He'd still have to explain why he didn't want Lily anywhere near her old friend

Parker.

She added milk to one of the mugs and discarded the used Keurig cups. Then she folded her arms across her chest and looked at him. "I'm listening."

Wolf blew out a breath. "The man's in love with you."

"What?" Lily blinked, then shook her head. "Don't be ridiculous. Parker's not into...I mean, he and I are friends. And I shouldn't have to keep justifying my friendship with him to you."

"If you don't believe me," Wolf said, "ask him. Tomorrow, when you drive down there. Go ahead and ask him, see what he says."

"I don't need to ask him anything," she said. "Parker is gay, all right? So he can't possibly be in love with me."

Wolf stared at her. "You're fucking kidding me."

"No, I'm not. I wouldn't joke about something like this."

He frowned. "How do you know he's gay? Did he tell you?"

"No, not exactly." She looked down at the untouched coffee. "I figure it's his business, and when he's ready to talk about, he will. His family's not exactly...progressive."

"So you've never discussed it with him? You just assumed because...what, you saw him with another guy?"

"Nick told me, okay?" She dropped her hands and glared at Wolf. "He said not to bring it up, because Parker still wasn't out to his family and it might make things awkward."

Awkward? Jesus Christ. This wasn't awkward. This was fucking unbelievable.

"Listen to me." He leaned forward and grasped her upper arms, making sure he had her attention. "Parker is not gay. Last week, when I came over and he was here? He went all territorial and basically told me to fuck off."

Her mouth fell open. "No way. That's not possible. He wouldn't say something like that."

"You think I'm making this up?"

"I *know* him. What you're saying doesn't make any sense."

He wanted to shake her. "Of course it does. The man

would give his right ball for the chance to get you in bed."

"That's ridiculous."

"What's ridiculous is thinking he's going to be satisfied forever with you throwing him the occasional contingency or pro bono case, while he leverages his contacts to help you spread the word that oh, yeah, doctors are people too." He leaned closer. "You want to know what else is ridiculous? It's me, waiting around on the sidelines, hoping like hell you'll finally cut him loose so we can all move on."

She stared at him, pale-skinned and wide-eyed, as his voice continued to climb.

"It's me—" his fingers tightened around her arms "— hoping you'll realize that it's not enough to fly in between speaking engagements for the occasional fuck, that what you and I have could be so much more, the real thing, two people who actually love and support each other no matter what. *That's* what's ridiculous."

For a moment, neither moved. And then he blew out a breath and released her.

She continued to stare at him. "But you…" Her voice faltered. She shook her head and stepped back, rubbing her arms. "You're the one who said you needed space."

"Yeah, I said a lot of stupid things."

She licked her lips. "I can't…"

"Lily—"

"No." She took another step back. "I'm sorry, but I can't do this."

"You can," he said, face tightening. "You just choose not to."

"I'm sorry."

He searched her face, hoping for…what? A softening of her expression? A tiny hint that maybe she might change her mind?

Sure. And maybe the heavens would open up and angels would start singing *Ode to Joy*.

Just because he'd done the unthinkable and fallen in love didn't mean Lily reciprocated his feelings.

"I'm sorry too," he said. He brushed a finger across Lily's cheek and then leaned in to drop a soft kiss on her lips. "Goodnight, Lil. I'll see myself out."

CHAPTER EIGHTEEN

It was a minor miracle that she managed to avoid getting into an accident on the drive down to San Diego.

During the meeting with Dr. Lee and her husband, Lily smiled and spoke in all the right places. But for the most part, she sat back and watched Parker interact with his new client.

She wasn't sure what she was looking for. Parker appeared the same as always. Dapper in a closely-fitted business suit with baby blue shirt and matching socks, silk tie, and polished wingtips, he exuded just the right amount of sympathy while still keeping the interview on track.

They left Dr. Lee's house several hours later with a legal pad full of preliminary notes.

"Lunch?" Parker said.

Lily nodded.

They settled on a diner within walking distance, where they were quickly seated in a red vinyl upholstered booth and left to study the laminated menu.

For once, Parker seemed more focused on Lily than the food. "That went well, don't you think?"

"Yes."

"Timin's not ideal," he said. "What with her bein' pregnant and all."

Lily blinked. "That was a joke, right?"

"You're not laughin'. I must be losin' my touch."

The waitress returned with ice water and coffee. "You folks ready to order?"

While Parker conferred with the woman over the mile-high sandwich options, Lily studied him. The blond hair that was just starting to recede. High cheekbones and thin blade of a nose. Deep-set gray eyes that met hers with a puzzled look when she didn't respond immediately to the waitress's repeated question.

Until yesterday, Lily would have sworn she knew him inside out. Now she wasn't so sure. Was it possible for Wolf, who'd met Parker only once, to recognize something she'd failed to see for years?

"All right," Parker said once they were alone again. "You been like a cat on a hot-tin roof all day. What's goin' on?"

"I'm trying to figure something out." She unfolded her napkin and smoothed it over her lap. "What's going to happen to your father's law practice after he retires?"

Parker laced his coffee with creamer and stirred. "That's still up in the air. Why?"

"You could move back home and take over. If you wanted to."

"Hypothetically speakin', I suppose I could." He tasted the coffee, then added more creamer. "'Course I'd need to pass the bar exam in North Carolina first, since there's no reciprocity with California."

"Sounds like you looked into it."

"Not since finishin' law school. But back then, sure, I was considerin' all my options."

"Why did you decide to stay here, instead of returning home?"

He pulled a couple fresh napkins from the metal dispenser at the end of their table and wiped a few drops of spilled coffee. "Well, I did have a job here. Don't know if you recall, I started out as an associate at Gordon & Rees."

"But you didn't stay there."

"No. A couple years was enough. I like bein' my own boss."

"Nick said you stayed because you were afraid your father would disown you if he found out you were gay."

Parker rested his spoon on a napkin before looking up at her. "He told you that?"

Lily frowned at his mild response. "Yes. So is it true?"

"Well, now, Asheville may not be San Diego, but my folks are pretty open-minded." He picked up the mug. "Besides, I like women too."

"You're *bi*?"

He took an unhurried sip. "Did Nick ever tell you the story of how we met?"

"You pledged the same fraternity."

"That was later," he said. "Before that, I tried to pick him up at Geisel."

Her eyes rounded. "No way."

"Mm-hm. I saw him a few times at the library, studyin' late. It was a Friday night, pretty deserted. I figured, why not? He was very nice about it. Turned me down, no hard feelin's. Later, when we were rushin' the same fraternity, he took me aside and told me not to worry, he wouldn't tell anyone what happened. Said he understood that I might not get a bid if the brothers knew I was a fag—" Parker raised his palm, stilling Lily's protest. "His words, not mine."

"I can't believe Nick said that. And you let him get away with it?"

His lips quirked. "I didn't set him straight, if that's what you're askin'."

"Why not?"

Parker dismissed her outrage with a careless wave. "He meant well. And he was a good guy. I liked hangin' out with him. Things were always more fun with Nick around. I'm not sure we would've become friends if he knew the truth."

"Why not?"

"Because in college it was all about getting laid. Sorry, darlin'—" he shrugged. "But that's the God's honest truth.

And for me, it was easier bein' the gay best friend than a competitor in the same dating pool."

"But what about later? Surely after college…"

"Nick went to med school, I went to law school. Different social circles. You know how it is. Life happens, you drift apart."

"But he still introduced you as his best friend."

"Yeah, that was Nick. Loyal to the end." Parker smiled and lifted his cup in a mock salute before finishing the rest of his coffee. "He came to my law school graduation, took me out to celebrate. And that's when he told me he'd met the girl he was fixin' to marry."

"Oh." Lily blinked. "But we didn't start dating until…"

"Later that year," Parker finished for her. "I know. Typical Nick, right? Once he made up his mind about somethin', that was it."

She and Nick hadn't met until their last year of med school, when Lily returned to clinical rotations after a year off to do her MPH. Up until then, she'd been a year ahead of Nick. And though they attended the same school, they might as well have been inhabiting two separate worlds—worlds that collided only when they were scheduled for the same fourth year clinical clerkship.

A year later, they both matched at UCSD. Nick in surgery, Lily in internal medicine. That's when they moved in together.

Parker set down his cup with a thump. "So there I was, slavin' away for Gordon & Rees, wonderin' if maybe Asheville wasn't a better option, when Nick called. Invited me over for dinner. I bought a nice bottle of wine, put on my Sunday best, and headed across town to meet my best friend and his girl."

"I remember that night," Lily said. "Nick got called in to the hospital because of some big accident on the I-5, and they needed as many hands as they could get in the O.R. And then you showed up, in your three-piece suit…"

"And we stayed up half the night, drinkin' wine and waitin' for Nick to come home. And when he did, do you remember what he said?"

She took a deep breath to ease the pressure in her chest. "Something about leaving me in good hands."

"Ironic, isn't it? I was a safe choice, 'cause as far as Nick was concerned, I was gay. If he knew what I was really thinkin', he'd have kicked my ass to the curb."

Don't ask. Do. Not. Ask. "What were you thinking?"

"That here's this amazin', smart, sexy woman—and Nick got to her first."

The waitress returned with their orders. "Here you go, folks. Enjoy."

Parker thanked her and reached for the hot sauce.

For several minutes they ate in silence. Then he sighed and wiped his fingers on a napkin.

"So now you know," he said. "The reason I stayed was because of you."

Lily frowned. "But...that's crazy. I was with Nick. You couldn't possibly believe I'd cheat on him."

"No." He sipped his water. "But Nick..."

"What about Nick?"

"Somethin' was off. He wasn't actin' like his normal self."

"He was sleep deprived," she said. "We all were. Sleep deprivation does crazy things to the brain."

"Yeah, maybe." He attacked the second half of his sandwich.

Lily watched him eat. "If you thought he was acting oddly, why didn't you say something?"

"I did."

"No you didn't," she said. "I would have remembered that."

"Not to you. To him. He brushed me off. Said the two of you were goin' through a rough patch."

"Oh." She drew a finger through the condensation on her water glass. "He told you that?"

"Yeah. So I backed off."

She pushed aside her barely touched plate. "It's true. We were. I was working hundred-hour weeks. Nick was logging a hundred and twenty. We hardly saw each other. And when we did…" She shook her head.

"I'm sorry," Parker said. "I was supposed to be his best friend, but all I could think was that if things didn't work out, you'd be free. It never occurred to me that he might be depressed. Or suicidal. When you called that mornin'…Jesus God, I wanted him out of the way, but not like that. Never like that."

She reached across the table for his hand.

They sat that way for a minute, hands clasped, not saying anything.

Lily finally stirred and sighed. "It never really goes away, does it? The guilt."

"No." He stared at their joined hands. "But seven years is a long time."

"I know." She gave his fingers one last squeeze and pulled away.

"I still think you're the smartest, most amazin', most beautiful woman I've ever had the pleasure of knowin'."

"Parker—"

"Please, Lily. We can make this work. We understand each other, respect each other. It's not just about Nick anymore. It about us, you and me—"

"I'm sorry, Parker, but I can't. You're a good friend. The best. I don't know what I would have done without you all these years—"

"I can be more. Let me show you. Just give me a chance, give us a chance."

"No, I'm sorry," she said. "You need to move on."

How many times had she heard those words? Said them to others? But she'd never truly owned them. Until now.

"You need to move on," she repeated more firmly. "And so do I."

Parker scowled. "It's him, isn't it?"

"Who?"

"That Wolf guy."

She hesitated.

"Listen to me, Lily. The guy's a prick. He doesn't

understand you, not like I do. And he has no regard for you or what you're tryin' to accomplish."

"You're wrong. It took him a while, but I think he finally gets it."

Parker's lips thinned. "You're makin' a mistake."

"I don't think so," she said. "But if I am, it's mine to make."

The waitress stopped by to top up their waters. "Anything more I can get you folks?"

Lily forced a smile. "Just the check, thanks."

The woman rifled through her pad and tore off a sheet, placing it face down on the table. "Here you go. You can pay at the register up front."

Lily and Parker both reached for the bill.

"My turn," Lily said.

They walked to the register together, and then retraced their steps toward the street where Lily had parked earlier.

"What about Sara Wiggs?" Parker said. "And Alicia Lee?"

Lily pressed the fob to unlock her car. "Tell me the truth, Parker. If we'd had this discussion years ago, would you have taken on their cases?"

He pursed his lips. "I don't know."

"But you won't abandon them now?"

"I'm not a quitter. The Wiggs case is practically settled, and I promise to do my best for Alicia Lee."

"Thank you."

"There's nothin' I can say to change your mind?"

She shook her head. "I'm sorry."

"We could've been good together."

She pressed a kiss to his cheek, then stepped back. "Take care of yourself, Parker."

"So this is it?"

She opened the car door. "After Alicia…maybe you should think about taking over your father's practice."

"Yeah," he said. "Maybe."

CHAPTER NINETEEN

The phone rang late Wednesday night, just as Lily was getting to the big reveal. She glanced at the screen. *Private number.*

Answer, or continue reading?

The ringing stopped, then started up again.

She sighed and sat up in bed, resting the book face-down atop the covers. "Hello."

"Lily?" a male voice said. "It's Doug Williams. Sorry to bother you."

"Oh, hi Doug. No bother."

"I have a favor to ask," he said. "There was an accident last night. You may have seen it on the news…"

"Wolf?" Her heart skipped a beat. "Oh, God, is he okay?"

"Uh, yeah. Far as I know. I mean, he's probably shaken up like the rest of us after hearing about it. Erik Harding, our chief of surgery, died. Crashed through a guardrail on the PCH and went over the side. It was a forty-foot drop, and his SUV landed upside down on the rocks. Apparently he wasn't wearing a seatbelt."

"Oh, no." Lily closed her eyes, relief mingled with dismay. "Was anyone else hurt?"

"No. He was alone in the car. No other cars involved.

Officially, the police are still investigating. But they think…" Doug hesitated. "I'm telling you this is in confidence, okay?"

"Of course."

"It looks like he might have planned this. He canceled his cases for the week, claiming a family emergency. But his wife, who's one of our ER docs, says she wasn't aware of any emergency. And the physical evidence suggests he didn't brake at all. The car was accelerating when he went over, though they won't know for sure until they download the black box data."

"Is there any way it could have been an accident? A malfunction of the brakes or the steering or something?"

"I suppose anything's possible," Doug said. "But they found a note in the glove compartment…"

"What did it say?"

"The police aren't releasing details yet. Just that there was a note, signed by Erik, addressed to his wife."

"I'm so sorry. The poor woman must be devastated." Lily drew up her knees and rested an arm across the top. "What do you need me to do?"

"Put together some kind of moderator-led discussion where hospital employees can talk about what happened. Provide some information about symptoms of burnout, tips on stress management, what resources are out there to help. I think it's especially important for those who didn't get a chance to attend the Postgraduate Assembly this year. Doctors, nurses, support staff. We need everyone to be more aware of the danger signs, so we can look out for each other."

"I can do that."

"And no sugar-coating," he said. "I'll clear it with Rachel—Erik's wife—first. But people need to know the truth. I'm not letting the administration sweep this under the rug."

"No," she murmured. "Of course not. What about grief counseling?"

"HR's working on it. There are a few local therapists who've helped us out in the past."

"Okay." Lily switched to speaker phone and pulled up her calendar. "When do you want to do this?"

"The next couple of days? Maybe two or three sessions, staggered so that everyone can attend at least one. I know it's short notice, but—"

"No problem." Lily slid out of bed and padded to the living room for her laptop. "Do you have a few minutes now? We can go over exactly what you have in mind."

So this was how it felt, when you discovered that the foundation on which you'd built your house consisted of nothing more than sawdust.

Wolf worked through the day's patients on autopilot, stopping periodically to repeat a heart or lung exam, or recheck his notes and orders, to make sure that even in his distracted state he didn't miss something important.

His cell phone pinged with a text reminder of the mandatory hospital staff meeting in the auditorium.

He was tempted to ignore it, until his eye caught the name at the bottom. *Speaker/moderator - Dr. Lily Reid.*

Damn. His chest hurt.

She'd talked about this.

Sometimes sucking it up wasn't enough. And the fittest didn't always survive.

He sat in the back, watching her. Listening to the familiar sound of her voice. If he closed his eyes, he could imagine that she was speaking to him alone. The words flowed over him, their meaning lost amid the turbulence of his own emotions.

The screech of the microphone brought him back to reality.

He slipped out of the auditorium while she was still taking questions.

For the rest of the day, his cell kept going off. One admission after another. He powered through them, perversely grateful for the reprieve from his thoughts. As long as he kept working, he wouldn't fall apart.

It was close to ten in the evening when he finally signed out. Instead of driving, he walked home, two and a half miles in the biting wind, head down, hands buried in his jacket pockets.

The following day, he bumped into Doug in the ICU.

"You look like hell," Doug said. "When's the last time you slept?"

Wolf shrugged. "I got a few hours last night. You?"

"It's tough." Doug frowned. "Who'd have thought? Erik, of all people."

"Yeah." Wolf rubbed the back of his neck. "How's Rachel? Have you seen her?"

Doug shook his head. "I heard she got admitted to L&D this morning. Thirty-three weeks, with preeclampsia. Christ."

"They're inducing her?"

"Not unless they have to. For now it's just a mag drip and some steroids. Tina's planning to stop by and see her later today." Doug glanced at his watch. "Lily's giving a talk in a few minutes. You coming?"

"I went yesterday." Wolf headed for the nearest computer station and logged in to check his patient list. "How many more talks is she doing?"

"This one, and a third one tonight at eight for the folks who couldn't make it during the day."

Wolf nodded. "I'll catch up with you later."

It was Friday night, and the turnout for her final session was larger than either of the previous two.

Maybe it was the venue—the large open-plan dining hall with its soaring ceiling and the prospect of food. Hospital catering set out a buffet-style spread of sandwiches, crudités, cheeses, fruit, and miniature pastries, along with a variety of non-alcoholic beverages.

But the atmosphere remained subdued, and much of the food went untouched.

"Good evening." Lily adjusted the volume on her portable microphone. "Can everyone hear me?"

She glanced around the sea of somber faces. "I'd like to thank you all for coming. My name is Lily Reid, and I've been asked to lead tonight's discussion about what we can do—both as individuals, and as a community—to help prevent future tragedies like the one that claimed Erik Harding's life.

"Before we get to that, though, let's all take a moment to reflect on the man whose death brought us here together. Some of you knew Erik as a colleague, a skilled surgeon, a friend, an esteemed leader in our community. He was also a son, a husband, a father.

"We've all had occasion to experience pain in our lives to varying degrees. Erik Harding was no different. What set him apart from the rest of us was his ability to hide that pain so well that no one around him saw his suffering.

"It's human nature to seek answers, particularly to existential questions that arise in the wake of tragedy. We want to know *why*. The problem is, we may never know what ultimately pushed Erik to take his own life."

A low murmur of voices rippled through the dining hall.

"What we *can* do," Lily continued, "is remember him, and all the other colleagues we've lost to suicide. And we can try to be more mindful of the challenges we face every day, more aware of how those challenges may affect us and our loved ones.

"So how do we do that? How do we learn to take better care of ourselves, to avoid getting burned out by all the responsibilities and pressures of our daily lives?

"And if we do get burned out, how do we recognize the symptoms in ourselves and others?

"And when we do recognize the symptoms, how do we deal with them, where do we turn?

"That, ladies and gentlemen, is what we'll be talking about today."

She noticed Wolf enter the dining hall halfway through her

opening remarks. He remained standing, leaning against one of the walls, a tall figure in scrubs and white coat, stethoscope draped around his neck.

By the time she wrapped up the Q&A, he was no longer there. A visual sweep of the room showed him heading toward the exit.

She hurried after him, weaving her way around clusters of people in scrubs of every color.

Wolf must have heard her approach, because he glanced back and stopped.

"Lily," he nodded. "Nice job back there."

"Thanks."

Up close, he looked like he was just coming off a three-day bender. Dark bags beneath red-rimmed eyes, stubble peppering his cheeks and jaw.

Several people passed by. Lily stepped out of their way.

"Are you done for the day?" she said.

"Pretty much," he said. "I was going to shower and change before heading out."

"Oh." She bit her lip. "Were you meeting someone?"

"Yeah. Stella Artois." He started walking again. "On tap at O'Briens down the street."

On tap? He was talking beer?

She rushed to catch up. "Can I join you?"

"Sure." He stopped in front of a door at the end of the hall and shot her a hooded glance. "I'll be out in five minutes. Unless you want to join me in the call room...?"

She licked her lips and looked around.

"Never mind," he said, removing the stethoscope from around his neck and stuffing it into his coat pocket.

Twenty minutes later, they were seated in a dark corner of the bar, Wolf with his lager and Lily sipping a hot chocolate laced with Kahlúa.

"He had everything going for him," Wolf said. "I mean *everything*. Busy practice. Wife and kids. They were expecting twins, for Christ's sake. What the fuck was he thinking?"

Lily cradled the mug in her hands. "Was there anything he

might have been worried about? A lawsuit? Family problems?"

Wolf frowned. "Everyone gets sued. That's why malpractice premiums are so high. As for family…I guess it's possible. I mean, he had an ex-wife and two kids in college, plus two more on the way. Maybe money…? Though that's hard to imagine. He had a thriving surgery practice. I bet he logged more hours in the O.R. than any other surgeon at St. Mary's."

Lily took a sip of her drink. "Maybe that was the problem."

"Too much O.R. time is a problem?"

Lily didn't say anything, just looked at him.

Wolf scrubbed a hand down his face. "Sorry."

She nodded. "Were you close?"

"We shared a lot of patients over the years. And Erik was the one who backed me up when I proposed starting a hospitalist program at St. Mary's. He went to bat for me with the medical staff." Wolf flashed a crooked smile. "Community hospital like this—you can imagine how much opposition there was to the idea. Took a while for the old guard to realize I wasn't taking business away from them."

"He sounds like a remarkable man."

"Yeah, he is. Was." Wolf signaled their waiter for a refill. "I still can't believe he's gone."

In the corner above the bar, a TV tuned to ESPN showed outtakes from some college football game. A collective groan went up from the crowd at the bar when the quarterback fumbled the ball.

Wolf glanced at them, then at Lily. "You think they realize they're watching a rebroadcast?"

She shrugged. "Sometimes that's better. You pick up details you might've missed the first time round."

The waiter exchanged Wolf's empty glass for a full one.

Wolf leaned back in his chair and stretched his legs out under the table, brushing Lily's calf in the process.

She shivered and closed her eyes.

"I guess I should apologize," he said. "For giving you shit about…everything."

She opened her eyes and met his gaze straight on. "Not everything. You did make the video, even if you didn't believe in the message."

"I wanted to get into your pants."

She had to smile at that. "You'd already done that. It wasn't a quid pro quo."

"I guess not." He raised a brow. "Maybe more of a love letter...?"

Something warm and fluttery settled in her belly. She took a deep breath. "I talked with Parker. You were right."

"Ah."

"I think he'll go back to North Carolina."

"I see." Wolf slowly straightened. "Where does that leave us?"

Her heartbeat sounded loud in her ears.

Could she take the risk? Open herself to the danger of loving someone, only to have it all snatched away? Not by depression or suicide—between Wolf's sense of humor and resilience, his solid support system of family and friends, and her own vigilance, honed over these last seven years—she doubted he'd succumb to those dangers.

But what if he simply changed his mind? Decided in a month, six months, five years from now that he'd made a mistake, and didn't want this relationship after all?

She'd be devastated.

And yet...she'd survive. Because she too had learned resilience. She was stronger, more confident now, living life on her own terms.

And the things she advocated for others—living in the moment, enjoying what was important, letting go of the rest—wasn't it time she started following her own advice?

Love and happiness were within her grasp. All she needed to do was reach out and say...

"Will you marry me?"

His mouth fell open.

"Kidding," she smiled. "How about we start with dinner at my place?"

"It's too late for dinner."

She glanced at the time. "You're right. How about ice cream?"

"Ice cream?" He blinked and stared at her, as if slowly coming awake from a dream. And then his lips turned up in a smile that warmed her to her very toes. "Absolutely. It's never too late for ice cream."

"We'll have to stop by the store to get some," she said. "I'm all out."

"My place is closer." He settled the bill and hustled her toward the door. "Plus I happen to have a few pints of chocolate salted caramel in the freezer."

She glanced at him, brows raised. "Pretty sure of yourself, weren't you?"

"Actually, no." He caught her hand and brought it to his lips. "But let's just say I was very, very hopeful."

~The End~

A NOTE FROM THE AUTHOR

Thank you for reading *The Burnout Cure*. I hope you enjoyed Wolf and Lily's story.

Readers always ask: where do I get my ideas? With *The Burnout Cure*, I didn't have to look far. While Wolf, Lily, and the characters who inhabit their world are fictional, the issues of physician burnout, depression, and suicide are very real—as are the sobering statistics that Lily quotes about how many physicians are affected.

The first seeds of this story were planted back when I was a young doctor-in-training. As Lily describes, the hours and work conditions were brutal. I lucked out with a residency program that provided wonderful role models and great institutional support. Unlike many of my peers, I didn't have to race from one hospital room to another throughout the night, drawing blood and starting IVs—our main teaching hospital had in-house phlebotomists and a great nursing staff who were paid to do that. But there were still entire months when I never saw the sun because I was pre-rounding on patients at 4:30 a.m., spending the day in the O.R., doing evening rounds on post-op patients in the SICU (surgical intensive care unit), and then signing out to the night team at 9 or 10 p.m.—when I wasn't on call myself. Speaking of call, I lucked out there too. I was never on call more often than every third night, and my longest stretch of working straight through without sleep was 42 hours. I had friends, though, who suffered through training programs like Nick's. They took call every other night, worked a hundred-plus hours each week, and lied to Joint Commission inspectors to keep their programs—and ultimately themselves—out of regulatory hot water for flouting the rules.

Fast forward ten years to another milestone event—or, more accurately, three milestone events—when three excellent, successful, well-respected physicians in our community committed suicide. Our local medical society held a dinner in their memory, and the keynote speaker talked about physician burnout.

I'd never heard about burnout prior to that night. But before long, the term seemed to be on everyone's lips. As Wolf notes in the opening chapter:

> *Whenever he opened a medical journal, or stepped into the doctors' lounge, or went to the ER to admit a patient, there was always someone talking about wellness, burnout, or both.*

Practically overnight, it seemed that physician burnout burgeoned to epidemic proportions, and even the popular press started quoting the grim statistics that those of us in the trenches lived with every day.

A few years ago, I came across a TEDMED talk by Pamela Wible, a family physician from Eugene, Oregon. She talks about "Why Doctors Kill Themselves"—and she doesn't mince words. She describes a broken system that dehumanizes aspiring physicians and perpetuates abuses in medical education and practice.

Dr. Wible's passion about the topic got me thinking.

What if a woman who is smart, mouthy, and willing to challenge the establishment decides to turn her personal tragedy into a cautionary lesson for other physicians? What if the one man who can help her spread the message is an irreverent, unapologetic chauvinist who doesn't believe in burnout? And what if they strike sparks off each other, hot enough to singe the mattress?

And so, *The Burnout Cure* was born.

Want to read more about this topic? Check out the bibliography on the next page, which includes citations for a few of the sources I found most helpful and compelling while researching the book.

BIBLIOGRAPHY

In Print:

Bernard, R. 5 ways to improve physician mental health. *Medical Economics*. 2017. http://bit.ly/2A52VBB. Accessed 24 Nov 2017.

Panagioti M, Panagopoulou E, Bower P, et al. Controlled Interventions to Reduce Burnout in Physicians. A Systematic Review and Meta-analysis. *JAMA Intern Med.* 2017;177(2):195–205.

Peckham C. Medscape Lifestyle Report 2017: Race and Ethnicity, Bias and Burnout. https://www.medscape.com/features/slideshow/lifestyle/2017. Accessed 24 Nov 2017.

Shanafelt TD, Hasan O, Dyrbye LN, et al. Changes in burnout and satisfaction with work-life balance in physicians and the general US working population between 2011 and 2014. *Mayo Clin Proc.* 2015; 90:1600-1613.

Sinsky C, Colligan L, Li L, et al. Allocation of Physician Time in Ambulatory Practice: A Time and Motion Study in 4 Specialties. *Ann Intern Med.* 2016; 165(11):753-760.

Wible, Pamela. *Physician Suicide Letters: Answered.* Pamela Wible, M.D., Publishing, 2016. http://amzn.to/2Av7plK

On the small screen:

Demania, Zubin. Are zombie doctors taking over America? *TEDMED talk*. https://youtu.be/QLqrjLBV95o. Accessed 24 Nov 2017.
Watch funnyman ZDoggMD (yes, he's a real doctor) talk about his journey from burned-out doctor to rappin' sensation.

Wible, Pamela. Why Doctors Kill Themselves. *TEDMED talk*. https://youtu.be/qyVAtZ9VZ4Q. Accessed 24 Nov 2017.

On the big screen:

Do No Harm. Exposing the Hippocratic Hoax.
A film by Robyn Simon.
http://www.donoharmfilm.com
Emmy Award winning writer/producer/director Robyn Symon teams up with Pamela Wible, MD in this 2017 documentary about physician suicide. Here is a synopsis from the project website:

> "Jumping off hospital rooftops, hanging themselves in janitorial closets, overdosing on drugs—they're A students and their suicides are often like well-planned school projects. Doctors are our healers, yet they have the highest rate of suicide among any profession. Medical students and families of physicians touched by suicide come out of the shadows to expose this silent epidemic and the truth about a sick healthcare system that not only drives our brilliant young doctors to take their own lives but puts patients' lives at risk too."

ABOUT THE AUTHOR

A native of Philadelphia, Jill Blake now lives in southern California with her husband and three children. During the day, she works as a physician in a busy medical practice. At night, she pens steamy romances.

To be notified when Jill has a new release, sign up for her newsletter at **http://eepurl.com/UMZZ9**

Jill loves hearing from readers!
You can contact her through any of the following:

Blog: http://jillblake.blogspot.com/
Facebook: https://facebook.com/jill.blake.3386
Twitter: https://twitter.com/Jill_Blake

ALSO BY JILL BLAKE:

<u>The Silicon Beach Trilogy</u>:
Beyond the Ivory Tower (Book 1) ~ Anna & Ethan
Sweet Indulgence (Book 2) ~ Becca & Leo
A Matter of Trust (Book 3) ~ Klara & Vlad

<u>The Santa Monica Trilogy</u>:
Without a Net (Book 1) ~ Eva & Max
Coming Home (Book 2) ~ Grace & Logan
Balancing Act (Book 3) ~ Angie & Zach

<u>Doctors of Rittenhouse Square Trilogy</u>:
Pursued by the Playboy (Book 1) ~ Kate & Marc
Taking a Chance (Book 2) ~ Samantha & Alex
This Time for Keeps (Book 3) ~ Isabelle & Luca

Turn the page to read more about these titles...

THE SILICON BEACH TRILOGY

Beyond the Ivory Tower *(Book 1)* ~ Anna & Ethan
When venture capitalist Ethan Talbot offers to pay top students to drop out of school, math professor Anna Lazarev goes on the warpath. But their battle over education takes an unexpected turn, thanks to a mutual attraction that's impossible to ignore.

Sweet Indulgence *(Book 2)* ~ Becca & Leo
Leo Kogan has a brilliant medical career, great friends, loving family. All that's missing is the perfect woman: Becca Markham. But going from friends to lovers proves harder than he expects—especially when Becca embarks on a risky business venture that threatens to turn Leo's safe, stable world upside down.

A Matter of Trust *(Book 3)* ~ Klara & Vlad
Venture capitalist Vlad Snezhinsky excels at two things: making money and being a dad. Still struggling through a bitter divorce, he has zero interest in romance—until he meets Klara Lazarev. But when murder throws their world into chaos, can new love survive when it's a matter of trust?

THE SANTA MONICA TRILOGY

Without a Net (Book 1) ~ Eva & Max
Betrayed by her husband, single mom to her young son, struggling to keep head above water, the last thing Eva needs is another philandering male. But when her best friend's older brother offers her a job, can Eva resist what may be the biggest adventure of her life?

Coming Home (Book 2) ~ Grace & Logan
Eight years after she leaves for New York, scandal sends Grace fleeing home and into the arms of her old college boyfriend. Sometimes, first love deserves a second chance—but can it survive when secrets and betrayals from the past come to light?

Balancing Act (Book 3) ~ Angie & Zach
When Angie goes head to head against her old nemesis Zach, "backroom negotiation" takes on a whole new meaning. As lawyers on opposite sides of a case, they've got plenty to argue about. But legal wrangling takes a backseat when their mutual attraction threatens to spin out of control.

DOCTORS OF RITTENHOUSE SQUARE

Pursued by the Playboy *(Book 1)* ~ Kate & Marc
A top-notch gynecologist with a playboy reputation, Marc DiStefano is finally looking to settle down. He sets his sights on Kate Warner, a career-driven woman who doesn't believe in love—and that's when the problems begin.

Taking a Chance *(Book 2)* ~ Samantha & Alex
When burnt-out family physician Samantha Winters trades her big-city career for a rural clinic, she figures it's a temporary gig. Falling for the local golden boy is not on her agenda. Alex Kane spent years building his company and raising his sister's orphaned kids. Now he's ready to cut loose and have some fun. Too bad the new doc isn't interested…or is she?

This Time for Keeps *(Book 3)* ~ Isabelle & Luca
When a senseless act of violence shatters her perfect world, Dr. Isabelle DiStefano struggles to rebuild: new life, new job, new man. But sometimes the past can be hard to let go of, especially when old flame Luca Santoro decides he wants her back…this time, for keeps.